# Dressing Matters

A handbook to help people with learning difficulties
to dress themselves

Philippa Moore DipCOT SROT

Illustrations by Jenny Valentine and Joan Henderson

Disabled Living Foundation

First published 1988

© The Disabled Living Foundation 1988
380-384 Harrow Road
London W9 2HU

British Library Cataloguing in Publication Data

Moore, Philippa
    Dressing matters.
    1. Mentally handicapped persons. Dressing – Manuals
    I. Title   II. Disabled Living Foundation
    646'. 31

ISBN 0-901908-50-9

# CONTENTS

|  |  | *page* |
|---|---|---|
| | Foreword | vii |
| | Acknowledgements | ix |
| | Members of the Steering Panel | x |
| | Introduction | xi |
| 1 | Teaching dressing: guidelines | 1 |
| | Assessing and teaching dressing skills | 1 |
| | Teaching other skills necessary for dressing | 16 |
| | Privacy | 21 |
| 2 | Teaching dressing: overcoming additional problems | 23 |
| | Delay in development | 23 |
| | Physical limitations | 24 |
| | Visual impairment | 26 |
| | Communication difficulties | 32 |
| | Limited hearing and vision | 35 |
| | Difficulties with attention and concentration | 39 |
| | Perceptual problems | 42 |
| | Lack of co-operation | 44 |
| 3 | Selecting clothes | 49 |
| | Encouraging choice | 49 |
| | Shopping | 54 |
| | Clothes for easy dressing | 56 |
| | Footwear | 60 |
| | Selecting 'safe' clothes | 62 |
| 4 | What affects clothes choice? | 64 |
| | Damage to clothes and footwear | 64 |
| | The need for protective clothes | 69 |
| | Physical factors | 74 |

5   Caring for clothing and footwear                          89
        Storing clothes                                       89
        Sewing and repairs                                    92
        Cleaning clothes                                      94
        Learning to care for clothes and footwear             97
        Caring for appearance                                 103

6   Financial assistance                                      107
        Sources of advice                                     107
        Allowances and grants                                 109

Appendix I:   Improving dressing skills: additional activities   114
         II:  Useful addresses                                   116

Index                                                          118

# FOREWORD

In our country everyone is normally dressed all the time. Dressing and clothing, and the suitability of clothes for the occasion, are a most important part of daily life; it is difficult to enter into education, employment or social life without acceptable clothing and footwear.

The ability to dress and undress unaided is an undervalued skill. For most of us, the struggle to acquire it is so far in the past that we take our ability for granted. Without it, however, independent living is impossible and only two courses are practicable. The first is to live in some form of residential care; the second, to have only a limited life, rising in the morning and going to bed at night not at the time preferred but at the time when those who can assist are available, or prepared, to help. If the carer is a family member, the carer's life and opportunity are similarly constrained. If the carer is a staff member, the costs of providing this assistance are substantial.

If independent dressing is impossible because of the degree of disability, the task of dressing can be a heavy and time consuming one, particularly if the person being assisted is severely disabled, or is incontinent.

Detailed information on the special clothing and dressing needs of people with learning difficulties seems to be sadly lacking, particularly their need for help in becoming independent, in selecting, purchasing, looking after and storing clothes and footwear. Until this book was written, no comprehensive information resource had been assembled for carers, despite the fact that wise choice of garments can do much to ease their task.

First impressions, which are vital for social acceptance, depend to a large extent on general appearance. For people with learning difficulties it is particularly important that they wear styles that ensure they are accepted into the community.

The Disabled Living Foundation (DLF) has sponsored projects on the important subjects of clothing and dressing for people with disabilities since 1963, and has for many years run a national Clothing Advisory Service, partly funded by the Department of Health. These projects have resulted in a large amount of resource material on clothing and footwear for disabled people. However, before *Dressing Matters* was researched and written, the DLF resources contained little information helpful to people with learning difficulties. The DLF Trustees were therefore very grateful when the DHSS agreed to fund the research and writing this book, and to produce further training material for carers. The Trustees thank the DHSS for this most important help and also for the advice and assistance given by their officers.

The research and writing have been guided throughout by a Steering Group whose members are listed on page x. The Trustees thank them warmly for their advice and for the time they gave to discussing the content of the book and the various drafts prepared.

The printing of *Dressing Matters* was made possible by a loan from King Edward's Hospital Fund for London, and the DLF Trustees are very grateful to the Fund which has assisted the Clothing Advisory Service in so many ways over the years.

The DLF Trustees were fortunate to find a dedicated project worker, Miss Philippa Moore DipCOT SROT, and hope that her enlightened approach to the many different aspects of her subject will be of use in a field previously so little researched.

We hope this book will be of assistance to people with learning difficulties and all those concerned in their care, both in improving skills, reducing work, increasing acceptability and in promoting the enjoyment and interest which most of us get from life through what we wear. The publishers would welcome further comment and advice on the book's content, so that its pioneering work can be developed in the next edition.

**W M HAMILTON**

# ACKNOWLEDGEMENTS

While working on this handbook, I have greatly appreciated the interest shown in the project and the advice offered by so many people. I would like to take this opportunity to thank all those people who have given me help and guidance while visiting schools, hospitals, social education centres, residential units, colleges, community teams and specialist advisory bodies, as well as the carers and professionals who have written to me with information and suggestions.

My thanks go to the members of the Steering Panel for their support and advice throughout the project and for the time they gave up to read and discuss all the draft manuscripts. I am grateful also to many other carers and professionals who have taken time to read and comment on the manuscripts, especially John Clements, Senior Lecturer in Psychology, Institute of Psychiatry, University of London.

I would also like to thank Peggy Turnbull MCSP, Clothing Adviser at Disabled Living Foundation (DLF) until September 1986, for her help and guidance when this project began, Janet Hughes MCSP for her valuable advice when planning the handbook and training pack, and Lady Hamilton CBE MA, DLF Chairman, and Elizabeth Fanshawe OBE DipCOT, DLF Director, for their support throughout the project.

I have greatly appreciated the help and advice from all the staff at the Foundation and am indebted to Debbie Sexton for tirelessly typing and retyping each chapter. I thank Ginny Jenkins MCSP, the present Clothing Adviser, and the staff in the Clothing Office of the DLF for their support and for the useful discussions I have had with them throughout the project.

I would also like to give my thanks to Joan Henderson and Jenny Valentine for illustrating this handbook, and to Diana de Deney for editing the text.

PHILIPPA MOORE

# MEMBERS OF THE STEERING PANEL

Lady Hamilton CBE MA, *Chairman, Disabled Living Foundation*

Mrs B Budd-Pickard MCSP, *Physiotherapist*

Miss M Collyer MChS SRCh, *Footwear Adviser, DLF*

Mrs E Cotton MCSP RG, *Vice Chairman, Conductive Education Interest Group*

Miss E Fanshawe OBE DipCOT, *Director, Disabled Living Foundation*

Miss B Godfrey DipEd, *Advisory Head Teacher, Inner London Education Authority*

Mrs A Gunner RNMH DipNurse(Lond) CertEd RNT, *Senior Nurse Tutor, Royal College of Nursing*

Mrs V Jenkins MCSP, *Clothing Adviser, DLF*

Mrs Gabi Michaelis MCSP, *Physiotherapy Adviser/Tutor, MENCAP*

Mrs C Ouvry DipEd, *Deputy Headmistress, Alexander Priory School, Inner London Education Authority*

A Parrish RNMH RCN, *Nurse Adviser Mental Handicap, Royal College of Nursing*

Mrs V Scarr FBCO DCLP DOrth, *Parent and Visual Handicap Adviser, DLF*

A K Shepherd RNMH CCDipTMHA, *Service Manager, Special Needs, Leavesden Hospital*

Mrs G Swain BD SRN, *Director of Nursing Services, Child Health and Mental Handicap, Leytonstone House*

Mrs C Tester DipCOT SROT, *Occupational Therapists' Special Interest Group in Mental Handicap*

**Observers**

Mrs P Gumery, *Procurement Division, DHSS*

Mrs J Pitts MA DipCOT, *Occupational Therapy Officer, DHSS*

K Pugsley SRN RNMH, *Nursing Officer, Mental Handicap Services, DHSS*

# INTRODUCTION

Getting dressed is, to some people, just a duty that has to be performed as quickly and with as little thought as possible; to others it is a pleasure to be relished. Whether we enjoy it or not, we all put on, take off and rearrange our clothing at regular intervals throughout the day. Without the necessary skills to get dressed, we are unable to choose when, how and what to put on and take off, and become dependent on others during this very personal activity.

By gradually building on each person's abilities and overcoming dressing and clothing problems in a way that fits in with the carer's own resources and time limits, this handbook aims to help all carers to encourage children and adults to become more independent when dressing, undressing, choosing and caring for clothes.

## How to use the book

The reader can either read the book from cover to cover or use it for reference. Chapter 1 should, however, be read first so that the general teaching guidelines it contains can be applied to the additional information in chapters 2 and 5. Each chapter ends with a list of further reading on specific subjects and, where possible, sources of further information – audio-visual material and advice services – on those subjects. Further Information on teaching skills (Appendix I) and some useful addresses (Appendix II) can be found at the back of the book.

## Terminology

To make reading easier, the person learning dressing skills has been referred to throughout the book as 'the learner', 'the wearer', 'a person with learning difficulties' and is taken to be male. For the same reason, while it is recognised that men and women have equal value in the caring and teaching role, the person teaching dressing skills is referred to as 'the teacher' or 'the carer' and is taken to be a woman.

# 1

# Teaching dressing: guidelines

To dress independently a person must be able to decide when to get dressed, be able to select appropriate clothing, recognise where each garment goes on his body and have the physical skills necessary to put the clothes on. If full independence is to be achieved, this process must take place with no supervision and no guidance. The skills necessary to increase independence in dressing and undressing can be taught to children and adults and, as each person's needs are different, teaching should be planned on an individual basis, working through the task in a systematic way.

Chapter 1 suggests how a teacher can break down this complex task into manageable parts. The reader should then be able to apply these guidelines to his or her own requirements and resources.

The first section deals with assessing and teaching the physical skills necessary for getting dressed, while the second concentrates on how to encourage discrimination skills and awareness of privacy.

The check lists set out in this chapter and in chapter 2 are merely illustrations of the type of lists that could be used. Since the strengths and needs of each person are different, it is important that a separate list to highlight those areas is made for each individual.

## ASSESSING AND TEACHING DRESSING SKILLS

### What should be considered before assessment and teaching begins

#### *Environment*

People rarely choose to get undressed or change their clothes in a place that is cold, public and unfamiliar; in order to encourage participation in dressing, therefore, the bedroom should be warm, private and familiar and, if possible, uncluttered and free from distractions. Screens and curtains can be used to ensure privacy and to block out distractions from outside and inside the room, but the teacher must make sure that there is still adequate lighting.

Furnishing should be considered at this stage. Those who prefer to dress sitting down will require a comfortable chair or bed that they can get on and off with ease. If they prefer to sit on the floor, a warm floor covering or carpet will make dressing more comfortable. Those who benefit from watching their progress while dressing and undressing will need to invest in a full length mirror.

Clothing should be stored in the dressing area in cupboards and drawers that are accessible both to the person getting dressed and the teacher.

## Summary

The dressing area should be:

- private

- warm

- comfortable

- uncluttered and free from distractions

- well lit

- suitably furnished.

## The assessor/teacher

Professional teaching skills are not needed to teach dressing; anyone who is interested and can identify a person's strengths and needs can break down the task and teach it stage by stage.

Teaching is often most successful if carried out by someone who is familiar to the person being taught, who recognises when help is needed but can also encourage independent progress. However, adults and children who have never had to dress themselves may find it difficult to accept that they must carry out the task with less assistance than usual. If this is so, progress may be slower if the teacher is a person whose role has previously been a purely 'caring' one, than if she is a less familiar person whose role is less clearly defined. The age and sex of the teacher may also affect progress, as some adults respond more positively to someone of the same sex and similar age who they can use as a guide to appropriate style and behaviour. The opportunity to choose such a teacher may be limited within a family and in some residential units.

An assessment of needs is usually subjective, even if a check list is used; if more than one teacher is involved, therefore, communication between them is vital when goals are planned and progress is recorded, so that the whole team is aware of the stage that has been reached, and of any changes made to an individual's routine. Everyone must work to the same aim and method.

It will usually take time for mutual trust and understanding to develop between teacher and learner. Some people may find it distressing to get dressed or undressed in front of a total stranger. The teacher must be aware of her own needs and limitations and, if necessary, seek help from other carers to make maximum use of her own and the learner's skills. New or unfamiliar carers should introduce themselves and give reassurance by communicating what is to happen through touch, gesture or the spoken word. It is also important that an unfamiliar carer finds out how each person communicates his needs.

Progress may be slow when teaching these skills; it is vitally important, therefore, that the teacher maintains her enthusiasm. A full understanding of the importance and advantages of increased independence should help to maintain a teacher's motivation.

## Summary

- Decide who is the best person to teach dressing.

- If there is more than one teacher there must be communication between all those involved.

- Mutual trust between teacher and learner is important.

- The teacher should be well motivated and be aware of her own limitations.

## The learner

To be receptive to learning new skills, the person being taught should be at ease and want to learn. If this is not the case, the teacher should try to discover whether anything (environment, time, teacher) can be altered to improve the situation.

Since any additional sensory handicap or physical condition will affect dressing skills, these should be recorded and taken into account during an assessment and when working out teaching priorities. Difficulties may arise if a person has not developed adequate control of his head, body or limbs; if muscle strength and joint movements in his arms or legs are limited, or if he has problems with manual dexterity or co-ordination. Sensory disorders, such as loss of hearing, vision, sensation or the ability to recognise and interpret information, will also affect a person's ability to learn; the teacher must consider whether the learner can understand what is expected of him, and can communicate his needs to her.

## Summary

- Look at the learner's attitude towards dressing.

- Look at learner's relationship with the teacher.

- Physical and sensory handicap must be recorded and taken into account when deciding which tasks to teach;

eg adequate control of  head
                                  trunk
                                  limbs

  adequate standing balance
                  sitting balance
                  joint mobility
                  muscle strength
                  grip
                  manual dexterity
                  co-ordination
                  vision
                  sensation
                  perception/recognition
                  hearing
                  communication skills.

See chapter 2 for adapting teaching techniques to meet these needs.

## Timing

The time taken to teach dressing skills is well spent, as the learner's resulting independence will leave direct carers more time for other activities.

All aspects of time should be considered when teaching dressing skills.

Each person must be allowed to get dressed in his own time while being assessed, and given help only when he cannot complete a task or becomes frustrated by it.

In the home a parent or carer's time may be unavoidably limited, but the length of time spent teaching a skill is not as important as how that time is used. It is often advisable to concentrate on one stage of dressing at a time, and to maintain the skills learnt during the first stage when work begins on teaching the next stage. Time will also be limited by each individual's capacity to concentrate; for those with a short concentration span, the

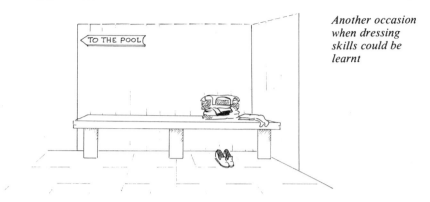

*Another occasion when dressing skills could be learnt*

teacher should again work on one stage at a time, as once the person being taught has stopped attending he will cease to learn.

Practising dressing skills should take place at an appropriate time of day; not only when getting up or going to bed, but also before and after other activities that require a change of clothes or extra clothes. To suggest that someone should get undressed and dressed again for no apparent reason can be confusing.

In residential units, routines and lack of staff time may interfere with dressing programmes. Staff in such units should examine their daily routine to see how assessment and the teaching of dressing skills can be fitted into it; they should look at the priorities of their residents: eg breakfast could be served later than usual; residents could have breakfast in dressing gowns and get dressed afterwards when staff are less busy; changing time before and after sports and outdoor activities could be extended to allow for dressing practice, and temporary timetables could be introduced with more activities requiring a change of clothes; dressing of the lower half of the body could be incorporated when using the toilet.

Successful teaching depends on both the teacher and learner being alert. If the person being taught is not at his best in the morning, for instance, it might be better if the teaching session took place at one of the alternative times mentioned previously. When the initial skills have been mastered at a suitable time for the teacher and the learner, it is vitally important that these skills are encouraged every time that dressing and undressing takes place.

## Summary

All aspects of time in relation to dressing must be considered:

- the amount of time allowed;
- the appropriate time of day;

- the time of day when the learner is most alert;
- the fact that skills learnt should be practised at all appropriate times.

## Clothing

Before dressing starts, the teacher should check that the wardrobe contains sufficient clothes of the correct size that are clean and in a good state of repair. When teaching the more complex skills of selecting clothes, the learner should be encouraged to check the contents of his wardrobe himself before getting dressed.

Clothes that are attractive to the learner can be a valuable motivator when learning to dress, and the teacher must consider what each person would like to wear when encouraging independent dressing.

Different items of clothing should always be stored in the same place in the cupboard/drawers so that they can be found easily.

### Summary

- There must be sufficient clothing.
- Clothes must be clean and in a good state of repair.
- Clothes must be of the correct size.
- The clothes must appeal to the wearer.
- Clothes must be accessible to wearer and teacher.

## Assessment

Before teaching begins, it is important to assess each person's dressing skills to identify their strengths and needs. The best way to do this is to watch the person dressing and undressing. A written list of the complete task broken down into small steps will help this exercise. If the carer writes down everything that happens when dressing takes place, she will be able to make a list covering all the relevant areas for each individual. Each step should have a space beside it so that the teacher can record what each individual does at each stage.

The amount of detail in each check list will vary according to the individual's ability. The teacher may choose to list each garment that is worn and record whether or not it was put on independently (See example I on page 7) or, if the learner fails to put on a particular garment, she may find it necessary to break the task down into smaller stages listing all the physical skills needed to put on that garment (see examples II and III on pages 8, 9). A more detailed breakdown will give a clear picture of the

*Example I: Getting dressed*

| Name | | | | |
|------|---|---|---|---|
| Date | | 3.9.86 | | |
| Puts on underwear | Pants | X | | |
| | Bra | X | | |
| | Tights | X | | |
| | Petticoat | X | | |
| Puts on over clothes | Skirt | X | | |
| | Blouse | ✓ | | |
| | Cardigan | ✓ | | |
| | Trousers | X | | |
| | Jersey | ✓ | | |
| | Coat | ✓ | | |
| | Shoes | X | | |
| Does up fasteners | Zip | ✓ | | |
| | Poppers | X | | |
| | Buttons | X | | |
| | Hooks | X | | |
| | Laces | X | | |
| Checks appearance | | X | | |

✓ = Completed independently
X = Cannot do this yet.

reasons for failure, which may be due to lack of knowledge of how it is done or lack of the physical skills necessary to do it.

The completed check list will enable the teacher to decide what to teach first and how it should be taught.

All check lists should be dated so that they can be used to record changes or progress.

## Teaching

If the carer finds that undressing is easier or more convenient to teach than dressing, she can teach this first using the same techniques, as undressing

*Example II: Putting on pants*

| Name | | | | |
|---|---|---|---|---|
| Date | 7·9·8 | | | |
| 1. Holds pants by waist elastic | ✓ | | | |
| 2. Lowers pants towards feet | ✗ | | | |
| 3. Puts first foot into leg hole | ✗ | | | |
| 4. Puts second leg into leg hole | ✗ | | | |
| 5. Pulls up to heel | ✗ | | | |
| 6. Pulls up to ankle | ✗ | | | |
| 7. Pulls up to knee | ✓ | | | |
| 8. Pulls up from knee to thigh | ✓ | | | |
| 9. Pulls up from thigh to hip | ✓ | | | |
| 10. Pulls up from hip to waist | ✓ | | | |

✓ = completes independently

✗ = Cannot do this yet.

encourages similar skills, is itself an important independence skill and is a good introduction to learning dressing. The teacher must decide what stage she is going to teach first and what teaching method she is going to use.

It is important to build on existing skills.

Example IV (see page 10) shows that, since this man can already pull up his pants from knee to waist independently, he must be able to grip his pants and pull upwards. The teacher should utilise this ability and encourage progress from that stage to stage 7. If, as in example V (see page 11), the learner cannot yet complete any stage without help, the teacher must decide whether she should start by teaching the first or last stages. She

*Example III: Taking off trousers with button and zip*

| Name | Date | 11·9·86 | | |
|---|---|---|---|---|
| 1. Grips waist band near button hole and button | | X | | |
| 2. Pushes button hole over button | | X | | |
| 3. Grips zip tab | | ✓ | | |
| 4. Pulls zip down | | ✓ | | |
| 5. Grips waist band | | ✓ | | |
| 6. Pulls trousers down — waist to hip | | ✓ | | |
| — hip to thigh | | ✓ | | |
| — thigh to knee | | ✓ | | |
| — knee to ankle | | ✓ | | |
| — ankle to floor | | X | | |
| 7. Removes left foot from trousers | | X | | |
| 8. Removes right foot from trousers | | X | | |

✓ = Completed Independently
X = Cannot do this yet

could begin by encouraging the learner to pick up his pants and lower them towards his feet independently giving him assistance with the last stages. In this way, as the first stage is learnt, the teacher will move on to the next step on the list, encouraging him to put his foot into the leg hole independently. Alternatively, the teacher may choose to concentrate initially on teaching the skills necessary to complete the task (pulling pants up from hip to waist) giving assistance with the first stages. In this way the learner will end

*Example IV: Putting on pants: showing some skills in last stages*

| Name | | | | |
|------|------|------|------|------|
| Date | 30·5·86 | | | |
| 1. Holds pants by waist elastic | × | | | |
| 2. Lowers pants towards feet | × | | | |
| 3. Puts first foot into leg hole | × | | | |
| 4. Puts second foot into leg hole | × | | | |
| 5. Pulls up to heel | × | | | |
| 6. Pulls up to ankle | × | | | |
| 7. Pulls up to knee | × | | | |
| 8. Pulls up from knee to thigh | ✓ | | | |
| 9. Pulls up from thigh to hip | ✓ | | | |
| 10. Pulls up from hip to waist | ✓ | | | |

× = Cannot yet do
✓ = Independent

the session on a successful note and, when that final stage has been learnt, the teacher could work backwards teaching each preceding stage in turn (ie pulling up to hip followed by pulling up to thigh and then pulling up to knee).

## Methods

Once the teacher has decided what stage should be taught first, she must find the best teaching method for each learner. When teaching dressing, guidance should be given to complete each task, and gradually withdrawn as the skill is learnt.

*Example V: Putting on pants: needs help at every stage*

| | Name | | | | |
|---|---|---|---|---|---|
| | Date | 10·5·86 | | | |
| 1. | Holds pants by waist elastic | X | | | |
| 2. | Lowers pants towards feet | X | | | |
| 3. | Puts first foot into leg hole | X | | | |
| 4. | Puts second foot into leg hole | X | | | |
| 5. | Pulls up to heel | X | | | |
| 6. | Pulls up to ankle | X | | | |
| 7. | Pulls up to knee | X | | | |
| 8. | Pulls up from knee to thigh | X | | | |
| 9. | Pulls up from thigh to hip | X | | | |
| 10. | Pulls up from hip to waist | X | | | |

X = Cannot yet do.

The guidance must be adapted to the learner's needs; initially, full physical help may be necessary to guide the learner's hands through the task, but this guidance should be less specific as the skill is learnt. Physical guidance may gradually be replaced by the spoken word, gestures or pictorial sequences in a book. It is the teacher's responsibility to decide which method is most effective; she should be aware that both too little and too much guidance will lead to a failure to learn and try to gauge the minimum amount of intervention needed for success.

Independence is achieved when each stage can be carried out consistently with no physical, verbal or gestured help from the teacher or any other person. When all direct guidance from the teacher has been withdrawn, some people may find that pictorial sequences in a book or inside the wardrobe door can be used as cues to maintain independent dressing skills.

*Example VI: Putting on pants: a record of guidance needed and incentives*

| Name | | | | |
|---|---|---|---|---|
| Date | 1·6·86 | 2·6·86 | 3·6·86 | 4·6·86 |
| 1. Holds pants by waist elastic | P | P | P | P |
| 2. Lowers pants towards feet | P | P | P | P |
| 3. Puts first foot into leg hole | P | P | P | P |
| 4. Puts second foot into leg hole | P | P | P | P |
| 5. Pulls up to heel | P | P | P | P |
| 6. Pulls up to ankle | P | P | P | G* |
| 7. Pulls up to knee | P | G* | I* | I* |
| 8. Pulls up from knee to thigh | I* | I* | I | I |
| 9. Pulls up from thigh to hip | I* | I* | I | I |
| 10. Pulls up from hip to waist | I* | I* | I* | I* |

G = Gestured help.
P = Physical help.
I = Independent
* = Reward given (praise and smiles)

## Incentives

If the teacher discovers that learning to dress independently is not rewarding enough in itself, she should provide incentives to progress that are attractive to the learner. Incentives must be given immediately and consistently following the successful completion of the task being taught.

The incentives used must be: attractive, appropriate to the particular person's age, readily available at the time and of short duration, so that the

*Example VII: Getting dressed: a record of strengths and needs*

| Name | | | | |
|---|---|---|---|---|
| Date | | 5·6·86 | 10·6·86 | 15·6·86 |
| Puts on underwear | Pants | ✓ | ✓ | ✓ |
| | Bra | ✗ | ✗ | ✓ |
| | Tights | ✗ | ✓ | ✓ |
| | Petticoat | ✓ | ✓ | ✓ |
| Puts on over clothes | Skirt | ✓ | ✓ | ✓ |
| | Blouse | ✓ | ✓ | ✓ |
| | Cardigan | ✓ | ✓ | ✓ |
| | Trousers | ✓ | ✓ | ✓ |
| | Jersey | ✓ | ✓ | ✓ |
| | Coat | ✓ | ✓ | ✓ |
| | Shoes | ✗ | ✓ | ✓ |
| Does up fasteners | Zip | ✓ | ✓ | ✓ |
| | Poppers | ✓ | ✓ | ✓ |
| | Buttons | ✓ | ✓ | ✓ |
| | Hooks | ✗ | ✗ | ✓ |
| | Laces | ✗ | ✗ | ✗ |
| Checks appearance | | ✗ | ✗ | ✓ |

✓ = Completed independently
✗ = Cannot do this yet.

learner understands what activity is being rewarded. In addition, the teacher should try and choose an incentive that will not disrupt the session, that can be either phased out when a skill is learnt without stopping the success it was rewarding, or continued indefinitely without inconvenience to the teacher or detriment to the learner.

Examples of incentives:

1. social – eg hugs, praise, smiles, pat on the back, squeeze of the hand.

This type of incentive is readily available and could be continued after a skill is mastered; however, it may not be sufficiently attractive to all learners;

2. food – small pieces that can be eaten quickly. While this type of incentive is attractive to many learners, it may not always be readily available in adequate quantities. Food may also cause problems to those on special diets or those who have a tendency to over eat or put on weight. It is also very difficult to withdraw this reward once the skill has been learnt without disrupting progress;

3. activities – eg music on radio/tape recorder, looking at a book. Activities can often be disruptive when used during a dressing session and will reduce concentration. Enjoyable activities following the session can be a powerful incentive as dressing or undressing may be the necessary preparation to join in those activities, eg getting changed for swimming, going to a party;

4. progress charts – that can be filled in, in sections, when each skill is mastered.
   These may be a useful incentive for children who can appreciate that the chart indicates their progress, and charts can be kept as a permanent reminder of their success. Charts are usually inappropriate for adults;

5. tokens, money, star charts – that can be saved up and used later to exchange for something the learner likes.
   This type of incentive, although readily available at the time, is only suitable for those who have the ability to understand that these can be exchanged for something that they want.

As each stage in a skill becomes a part of everyday life, the incentives should be withdrawn gradually and used to encourage success in the next stage.

## Recording progress

A record of progress made is essential to guide the teacher in deciding what to teach next; it can also motivate both learner and teacher. Records show which dressing skills have been mastered and also how often and what type of incentives were used. The teacher must decide how often to record progress. If more than one teacher is involved, daily records may be necessary as it is vital to keep everyone who is involved up to date with progress and any alterations in the programme (example VI, page 12). Others may prefer a more general chart that can be used as a long term record of progress, once a week or once a month, indicating when the learner has mastered a particular skill and completed it consistently (example VII, page 13).

Ticks and crosses are a quick and simple way of recording strengths and areas of difficulty (example VII, page 13), but the teacher may find that a simple code system (example VI, page 12) using letters or symbols will be just as quick and give more information. If code systems are used, an explanation of each symbol must be kept on each record sheet.

Records must be easily accessible for reference and for updating, but preferably not on display for everyone to see. Carers may find a suitable place to store records of progress in the learner's bedroom; they could be kept inside the wardrobe door or inside a bedroom drawer.

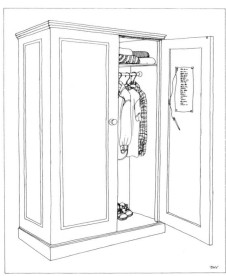

*Record of progress kept inside wardrobe*

## Summary: assessment, teaching and recording

Carers should:

● find out and record each individual's strengths and needs;

● decide what skill to teach first, taking into account all the surrounding circumstances;

● find out what is the best form of guidance for each individual;

● discover the most suitable incentive to encourage learning;

● monitor the amount of guidance given at each stage;

● monitor the effectiveness of incentives;

● keep written records of progress;

● make changes when a skill has been learnt, or when no progress is being made and a different approach may be more successful.

# TEACHING OTHER SKILLS NECESSARY FOR DRESSING

As well as mastering the basic skills needed to put clothes on and take them off, some people may be able to learn *what* clothes to put on, *where* to put them on the body, and to differentiate between the front and back of each garment and *whether* or not it is inside out. The ultimate aim is that each person should decide for himself what is appropriate to wear each day, and how it should be worn.

Methods of encouraging these discrimination skills are listed below.

## How to teach where, and in what order, clothes should be worn

### When storing clothing

Those who find it difficult to identify which item of clothing is worn on which part of the body could store different garments in separate areas of the cupboard/drawer.

Picture labels on cupboard doors could be used showing each garment on the appropriate part of the body.

### When dressing

In the early stages, one of each garment should be laid out on the bed/chair in the order they are put on. When the learner has begun to put on all

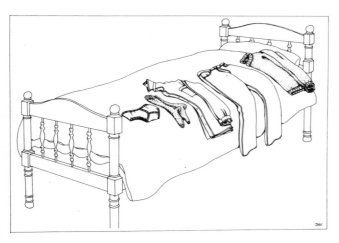

*Garments laid out before dressing*

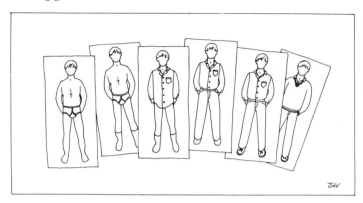

*Picture sequences to show the order in which clothes go on the body*

clothes in the correct order, the teacher could start changing the layout and then try putting out more than one of each garment. Later on, all garments could be left in the wardrobe.

Each item of clothing should be named while dressing, and the part of the body it goes on should be pointed to or touched as the garment is put on.

A mirror could be helpful so that the learner can see the garment before and after it has been put on.

Picture sequences in a book or wall chart can be used to show the order in which clothes go on the body.

## During other activities

Repetition is vital if this skill is to be learnt. Activities to improve knowledge of body parts will help this skill to develop. Learning about the different parts of garments can be reinforced when washing, ironing and folding clothes.

## How to teach which way round clothes are worn

### When storing clothes

Clothing that is returned to the cupboard/drawer must always be turned outside out and folded uniformly.

### When selecting clothes

Clothing which has a clearly defined front and back, inside and outside, will be helpful when teaching this skill, eg patterns, colours, seams, pockets (see page 57).

Clothes could be chosen with fasteners in the same place (eg all zips and buttons at the front).

Markers and labels sewn in the same position in all garments can act as cues to back and front, inside and outside (existing labels can be added or re-located).

## When dressing

Initially, clothes should be laid out on the bed or held up in the same way each day so that they can be picked up and put on without being rearranged. Later, when progress has been made, they should be left in the cupboard.

The learner needs time and encouragement to look at each part of the garment and locate important features, such as the head hole and armholes, before starting to put it on.

He should be encouraged to hold clothes up against his body before putting them on.

Mirrors should be used for self appraisal after putting on each garment.

The learner should be encouraged to check that each garment feels right when he has put it on.

## Choosing clothes to suit the weather and activity

Everyone should be given the opportunity to choose what clothes they like to wear, but some may need guidance as to which clothes are appropriate for each day (see chapter 3 for style, age-appropriate clothes and the importance of choice).

## When storing clothes

Organising the wardrobe is very important; extra space or divisions may be necessary. Summer and winter clothes should be kept in different areas as should everyday wear and clothing for special activities, eg work clothes, sports clothes.

Labels on the outside of the cupboard or drawer can illustrate what type of clothing is inside (these could be cut out of magazines). Alternatively, photographs of the learner engaged in different activities could be used. The teacher must find out which method of labelling is most helpful to each individual.

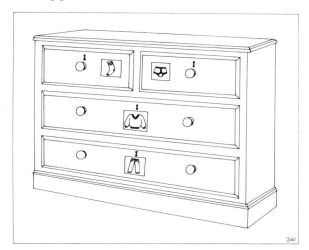

*Labels on drawers illustrating what type of clothing is inside*

## When selecting clothes

Each day appropriate reminders should be given about what will be happening and what the weather is like; the learner should look and feel outside the window or listen for rain and wind.

A carer could show the learner what *she* has chosen to wear depending on the weather and the particular activity.

Different fabrics and garments should be felt and tried on to find out how warm or cool they are.

Each person should be given plenty of time to make his decision.

## When dressing

Items of clothing that have been selected could be felt, looked at and talked about to decide if they are suitable or not.

The learner should be allowed to make mistakes so that he can learn from his own experience. Extra time may be needed in the early stages for the learner to correct his mistakes.

Self appraisal in a mirror is important.

## During other activities

The learner should be encouraged to look at what others are wearing – in magazines, on the television, in shops, outside and during different day-to-day activities.

## Distinguishing between clean and dirty clothes

### When storing clothes

When undressing, encourage each person to put underclothes into a laundry basket ready for washing.

All outer clothes should be checked individually by looking and by smelling, and those that are dirty put into the laundry basket straight away. Any clean clothes should be returned to the cupboard/drawer in the usual place.

### When selecting clothes

Removing clothes from the laundry basket should be discouraged by ensuring that clean, well fitting clothes that are attractive to the learner are in the cupboard/ drawer.

Each item chosen from the cupboard should be looked at and smelt to convince the learner that it is clean.

### When dressing

A routine of changing clothes every day, or after each bath, may help some people to make the distinction between clothes that need washing and clothes that are ready to wear.

Self appraisal in the mirror, checking that clothes look clean and ironed, should be encouraged.

The teacher should make it clear to the learner how he looks.

### During other activities

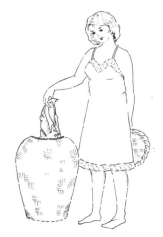

When possible, each person should be involved in the washing process, or at least be aware that it happens (see page 97). The difference between clean and dirty clothing can be emphasised more strongly if they are seen and smelled before and after the washing process. If the learner is to be aware of potential dirty or smelly areas of his clothing it is essential that he understands something about the way in which the parts of the body function.

*Dirty clothes should be put into the laundry basket each evening*

The difficulties encountered when teaching these discrimination skills are many and varied. When these skills have been taught successfully and no assistance is required, an organised and consistent storage system for clean clothes and those garments that need washing will help to maintain independence (see page 89).

## PRIVACY

Privacy is something that most people value, especially where personal activities, such as getting dressed and undressed are involved. For those who rely on help from other people during these activities or who are learning dressing skills, it is important that the carer/teacher respects their right to privacy. Everyone has different standards of privacy and we cannot impose our standards on others; it is, however, important that people understand what is, and is not, appropriate when they are out in the community.

It is essential that teenagers and adults who have learnt dressing skills should understand that there are appropriate times and places for being clothed and naked. The importance of privacy is difficult to teach, but we can learn by seeing how others behave both in public and in private, and from other people's reaction to nudity. Carers should talk about the importance of privacy in different situations and should decide on an appropriate approach to this issue. Sex education could incorporate the importance of privacy and this can be reinforced by a consistent reaction to inappropriate nudity. A carer should always knock on the bedroom or bathroom door before entering, and ask if everyone is dressed and if they mind her coming in. If someone is undressed or not sufficiently dressed when a carer enters the room, she should go out again, explaining that she will be back when that person is decently dressed. This consistent attitude towards privacy may be the only way of instilling some idea of its importance.

## FURTHER READING

Carr, J *Helping your handicapped child.* Harmondsworth, Penguin, 1980.

(explains to parents and other carers how tasks can be broken down and taught to children)

Carr, J and Yule, W eds., *Behaviour modification for the mentally handicapped.* London, Croom Helm, 1980.

(an introduction for nurses and other professionals who wish to use behaviour modification as a method of teaching skills)

Jeffree, D M, et al. *Teaching the mentally handicapped child.* London, Souvenir Press, 1977.

(a guide for parents and other direct carers on teaching skills)

Popovitch, D and Lahan, S. *The adaptive behavior curriculum. Volumes I and II.* Baltimore, Paul Brooke Publishing, 1981.

(a comprehensive guide for nurses, professionals and carers, that breaks down basic and advanced dressing skills for teaching)

# 2

# Teaching dressing: overcoming additional problems

Some people with learning difficulties have additional problems that affect their dressing skills and ability to learn.

Chapter 1 sets out the general guidelines while this chapter contains more specific information to help those with particular problems to improve their dressing skills.

In this chapter each problem is dealt with under a separate heading, so that carers trying to help someone with a number of difficulties will find ideas in each relevant section.

## DELAY IN DEVELOPMENT

People are not born with the skills needed for dressing, and anyone learning to dress must be given the time and opportunity to develop the necessary controlled body movements and co-ordination. The learner will need to have some control of head and body so that a well balanced position can be maintained while dressing. To put on and remove clothing, controlled movements of the whole arm and leg are necessary as well as fine movements of the hand. Once these physical skills have developed they must be co-ordinated so that activities can be carried out unaided.

The carer will not be able to teach dressing until the learner is developing the necessary physical skills to apply to that task.

Each person develops at a different pace, and delay at one stage of development will affect the acquisition of dressing skills.

Advice should be sought from physiotherapists, occupational therapists, nurses and teachers on how the learner can be encouraged in these skills as they develop when he is dressing and also when involved in other activities.

It takes several years for any child to develop the physical abilities needed to get dressed. The carer must always be aware of each person's limitations and take advantage of any abilities he has, giving guidance rather than assistance as each skill develops.

## Summary

- There are several stages in the development of full physical function.

- Each person's rate of development is different, and delays may occur at any stage.

- Help can be sought from professionals to encourage development in any area where there is delay.

- Dressing skills can be mastered as the learner develops the ability to move, co-ordinate and control his body.


## PHYSICAL LIMITATIONS·

Learning dressing skills can be affected by physical conditions that lead to limited strength, muscle tone, range of movement, balance or co-ordination. The carer must consider each individual's needs and abilities, giving him the opportunity to participate as much as possible in the dressing process. Occupational therapists and physiotherapists should be contacted through social services or health service community teams to give advice on overcoming specific physical problems when teaching dressing skills.

### Environment

A person with physical limitations needs to be relaxed if he is to make the most of his physical abilities; to encourage his involvement in the dressing process it is therefore very important that it takes place in a warm, comfortable, 'safe' environment. (See also page 1.)

### Positioning

To encourage someone to take an interest and participate in dressing, the carer must consider all the options before deciding which is the best dressing position – the learner must feel confident, have some freedom of movement and a good view of what is happening: he could sit on a chair, on the floor, on the bed, or on a stool, with support at different levels. Those who have difficulty getting dressed while supporting their bodies in an upright position may find lying on the side, front or back preferable. Propping up the head with pillows, or using mirrors will often help those who get dressed while lying down to see what is happening. If someone prefers not to use mirrors during dressing, however, this wish should be respected. People with increased muscle tone must be positioned carefully so that their tendency for tight muscle patterns, which greatly restrict free movement, is avoided. Advice should be sought from occupational therapists and physiotherapists to ensure that the chosen position is not impeding function, or encouraging fixed deformities.

## Lifting

The needs and preferences of the person being moved should be considered when a suitable method of handling is being sought, and the carer should be taught to lift without damaging herself or the person getting dressed. Physiotherapists can give advice on safe lifting techniques, and photographic or diagrammatic reminders can be helpful. Confident (not hesitant) handling will reassure the person getting dressed. It is important to warn the learner of any handling or lifting so that he is prepared for it.

## Timing

If the person getting dressed has limited strength and stamina, the teacher may choose to restrict his contribution to dressing to conserve his energy for other activities during the day. Time can still be spent on non-physical tasks, eg choosing clothes. (See also pages 4 and 49.)

## Choice of clothes

Choosing clothes is one way in which a person with gross physical limitations can become involved in the dressing process. The carer should encourage him to help select his own clothes so that his preference for styles and colours becomes apparent (mirrors can be used for self appraisal). Those people whose physical limitations make it difficult for them to speak may be able to make their preferences known through facial expressions or eye movements (see page 32 for difficulties with communication and pages 56 and 86 for clothes that are easier to put on or remove). (See also page 6.)

## Recording

Written records are important, especially if more than one carer is involved, to ensure that methods of lifting, positioning and the level of each person's physical involvement are monitored. (See also page 14.)

## Other activities

Movements related to dressing can be practised at other times in the day to help build up tolerance, confidence, strength and flexibility. Physiotherapists should be consulted about suitable exercises.

## *Summary*

- Help should be sought from professionals to overcome specific physical problems when teaching dressing.

- Each person should be given the opportunity to use their existing physical, intellectual and sensory skills while dressing.

- The most suitable position for each individual must be found to encourage them to use their skills.

- Inappropriate lifting and handling techniques could lead to loss of confidence and physical damage.

- Other activities can be used during the day to encourage dressing skills.


## VISUAL IMPAIRMENT

A person with a visual impairment as well as a learning difficulty will need careful teaching to enable him to understand his environment, learn about his body and improve his independence in all aspects of life. Someone who can see, can watch how others get dressed, what they choose to wear and how they react to what others wear, even before formal teaching of dressing skills begins. A person with a visual disability does not have these clues and must rely on touch and on all the other senses and powers of reasoning to learn. Teaching must therefore be well structured, consistent and make the maximum use of each individual's skills and abilities. Observation by carers is important to find out how each person's skills are affected by their visual impairment. Assessment of vision by an ophthalmologist is also important to find out the nature of each person's visual handicap, and how much residual vision they have. Technical officers for the blind, employed by some social service departments, can give detailed advice on teaching methods, and help carers to organise the environment and lighting to enable the learner to use his residual vision and other senses to the full. Knowledge of the nature and extent of his visual handicap will help staff to gear their expectations of performance at the right level. Carers may be over protective of people who have visual handicaps because, understandably, they fear accidents if exploration or experimentation with self-help skills is allowed. Too protective an attitude leads to a lack of opportunity to practise skills, and carers' low expectations may lead to failure to learn.


## Selection of clothes

Special clothes are not necessary for people who have a visual disability, but careful thought when selecting style and fabric can often help when teaching dressing skills and when encouraging interest in clothing.

## Style

A selection of clothes in simple styles with no fasteners (or one fastener only in the same position on each garment) would make dressing easier in the early stages. Those who have learnt to identify clothing and have mastered basic dressing skills should be free to choose whichever style they prefer. Styles with a clearly defined front and back will give cues to the person who is learning to position their clothing correctly, and this definition can be made in many ways (see page 57).

When basic discrimination between different types of garment has been mastered, the learner may be able to choose styles and colours that he wishes to wear. The carer should take notice of what styles he feels most comfortable in, and tell him what looks attractive (even if you cannot see yourself, it is important to know how you look to other people). Carers should make it clear what colours suit the person getting dressed and give constructive criticism when mistakes are made. This is the only way that a person with a visual handicap can learn what suits them best. To avoid colour clashes when choosing clothes each day, clothing bought could be limited to a selection of matching or co-ordinating colours and patterns that suit the wearer. Those with residual vision must

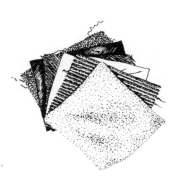

*Each person will prefer different fabrics*

be encouraged to use their vision to its best advantage; mirrors with appropriate lighting should be used to check colours and styles.

## Fabrics

As touch is so important to people who have a visual handicap, the 'feel' of different garments must be considered when selecting clothing. Fabrics chosen should feel comfortable when worn against the skin and each person will have their individual preferences. Accessories, such as belts or pockets and textured patterns in the garment, are useful identifiers, and may encourage an interest in clothing and dressing. However, too many textures on one garment may cause confusion when dressing skills are first being taught.

## Footwear

Narrow, high heels should be avoided by people who have a visual disability as a stable walking base is important to increase confidence and encourage independence when moving about. Broad-based heels of no more than 2 inches high, with a non-slip sole, will give a good base when walking.

## Storage of clothes

When first teaching dressing skills the carer will probably hand each item of clothing to the learner in turn, or lay each garment out flat on a table in front of the learner (or on the bed) with fastener undone and openings facing the right direction. In this way each garment can be felt and explored individually, and concepts of size and shape can be understood before it is put on. In time all the clothing may be laid out in this way at the same time and the learner should then be able to distinguish between different garments through touch before putting them on. As the learner's knowledge of garments increases, they can be left folded (in the same way each day) either individually or in a pile for him to identify and place appropriately on his body. The learner may then progress to selecting his own choice of garments from more than one of each left out on the bed or table and, in time, begin to select clothing from the wardrobe.

To make selection from the wardrobe easier, consideration must be given to the organisation of storage.

1. Identification – in a shared room each person's wardrobe must be identifiable; it can be labelled if necessary with an easily recognisable texture on or near the handle (eg a strip of furry fabric stuck on to the door, silky ribbon tied to the handle).

2. Space – a spacious wardrobe is necessary so that garments can be easily identified.

3. Organisation – clothes must always be put away in the same place and folded in the same way. Dirty clothes must be put in the linen basket immediately after removal and clean clothes put back into the wardrobe. All hangers could be hooked onto the bar in the same direction and hangers not in use should be taken off the bar and left on a shelf or in a bag until needed again. Hangers can be used for one garment only – or matching separates can be hung together. Socks and stockings should always be kept folded in pairs.

4. Divisions – maximum use must be made of all drawers, shelves, hooks and racks, so that clothing can be divided up in a way that suits the individual's needs and abilities, eg all socks or pants in one drawer; all colour matched garments on one shelf.

To improve wardrobe facilities, see page 90.

## Environment

When initially teaching dressing to a person who is visually handicapped, a chair that supports the learner at the back and at both sides with his feet flat on the floor will give total support so that his concentration can be focused on feeling clothing, listening to instructions and carrying out the tasks required to get dressed. Sitting on the floor leaning against a wall will give similar stability. (See also page 1.)

If clothing is to be laid out on a table in front of the chair it should be at elbow height so that the person getting dressed can explore the surface of the table with ease. A raised lip added to the edge of this table will help to prevent clothing sliding off and provide a boundary for exploration.

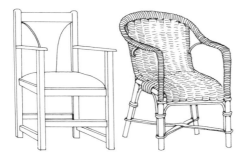

*Chairs that give support*

If possible, distractions which may prevent someone with visual handicaps from paying attention to the dressing task should be removed from the room. People with some useful vision may be distracted by bright colours, patterned wallpaper and nearby objects; this problem can be overcome if the clothes they are locating stand out against a plain background. Tactile distractions should also be kept to the minimum in the dressing area. Careful observation of the learner during dressing may help to identify distractions not immediately obvious to anyone with full vision. Sounds made by other people nearby may distract the learner and should be excluded when possible. Furniture and essential objects in the dressing area must be kept in the same place during teaching sessions, so that the environment remains unchanged while the learner explores garments and learns new skills.

## Assessment

Since a person who is visually handicapped will obviously find it difficult to master steps in the tasks that require vision, the task breakdown must be individually designed to take account of all possible areas of difficulty. (See also page 6.)

## Routine

A uniform method of teaching dressing skills is important, and, when more than one carer is involved, they must all make sure that they are teaching in the same sequence so that the learner is not confused. When basic skills have been learnt step by step, skills should also be practised in all appropriate situations and environments.

## Timing

Plenty of time must be allocated for the learner to study each garment – its shape, texture and where it goes on his body. This involves learning about the different features of each garment; identifying sleeves, collars and waistbands, for example, by touch or vision. Learning this skill cannot be hurried and, to make sure it is acquired, carers with little time could limit dressing each day to one type of garment and only progress to the next garment when the first is familiar to the learner. (See also page 4.)

## Guidance

Verbal instructions should be clear and simple, and all those involved in the dressing routine should use a uniform vocabulary. Physical help to guide

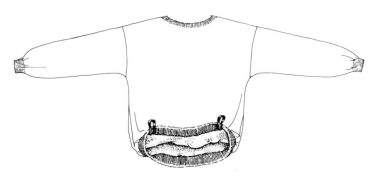

*Loops to identify the waistband of a jersey*

the learner's hands through the task is often necessary. When giving such help the teacher may stand in front of, or behind, the learner (see page 36) depending on which position is most acceptable to him. (See also page 10.)

## Positioning clothing

Distinguishing labels on clothing can be used to check whether it is on the right way or to identify the waistband of jerseys, 'T' shirts and pants when the garment is put on. When clothing that has a clearly defined front and back is used (see page 57) the learner will need initial physical guidance to enable him to learn about a garment's distinguishing features and to relate these to the part of the body it covers. Such guidance will be reduced as the skill is learnt. (See also pages 16-18.)

## Clean and dirty clothes

A person who is visually handicapped must be encouraged to make maximum use of his sense of smell and touch to discover if clothing is dirty or stained. The carer must encourage exploration of each garment, morning and evening, and teach the wearer to locate areas that are likely to smell or be stained. Checking for food stains after meals is also important. When a visually handicapped person is able to take responsibility for deciding what is clean enough to wear each day, carers should still draw his attention to undetected clothing stains. (See also page 20.)

## Checking appearance

Feedback on overall appearance is very important for those who cannot see for themselves. When clothing has been selected the learner must be encouraged to feel for untucked shirts and undone fasteners. Hair should be felt before and after brushing so that the difference can be recognised. Those with residual vision must be encouraged to look in a well-lit mirror to check their appearance.

## Other activities to improve dressing skills

Every opportunity must be taken during the day to practise dressing skills so that the tasks become familiar outside the strict routine established in the morning and evening. By touch and physical contact with other people through exercises a person with a visual handicap will learn how other people's bodies move and relate it to his own. Increased knowledge of his own body, its range of movement and limitations in the environment will give him more confidence when carrying out self-help skills. A person with a visual handicap will use his feet and finger tips to explore his environment. Movements of the whole body will improve balance and confidence when walking. Activities that improve fine finger movements and encourage touch and exploration with finger tips will improve the function of the hand and make it a more useful tool in self-help skills.

Some schools or day units may find that a session during the day can be allocated to people learning about their bodies or clothing. Shopping for clothes, washing and ironing them or sorting laundry piles are all useful activities to help a person with a visual handicap to become more familiar with different garments.

## *Summary*

- A person with a visual handicap does not have the same opportunities for incidental learning as someone who can see.

- An assessment is important to find out how much vision is retained.

- Tactile clues on garments will make selection easier.

- Storage of clothing can be organised to make selection easier.

- When teaching – all tactile and auditory distractions should be excluded.

- A set routine is valuable.

- A carer should encourage a person with a visual handicap to explore, so that he understands his body and his environment.

- Feedback from carers and companions is vital.

# COMMUNICATION DIFFICULTIES

Two-way communication when dressing is important to establish trust and to help the person getting dressed to understand what is expected of him and what is happening. Difficulties with communication can be caused by deafness or a limited ability to understand or use the spoken word.

## Assessment

Before dressing skills can be assessed or taught, the carer must first find out the nature of the communication difficulty and whether it is caused by limited hearing, limited physical ability to speak, a delay in the development of language, poor understanding of language, poor memory for language or poor attention, and then discover the best way to communicate and compensate for these problems. Professional help should be sought – a speech therapist can give an appropriate language assessment and an audiologist a hearing assessment (contact the local speech therapist and audiologist through the GP, health centre or hospital). (See also page 6.)

## The teacher

Whoever teaches dressing skills to a person who has communication difficulties must make sure that she knows just how much that person understands. She must be prepared to use visual cues, eg signing, pointing or miming, to help him to understand and to encourage him to communicate his needs. The teacher's approach must be consistent, and once the most effective level of communication has been found, it should be maintained – full advantage being taken of any progress made beyond that basic level. The teacher needs to communicate not only to pass on skills but to encourage the learner to trust her and co-operate with her; tone of voice and facial expression may establish trust and encourage co-operation. (See also page 2.)

## Environment

If possible all visual and auditory distractions should be excluded from the dressing area. The room should be well lit and arranged so that teacher and learner can communicate face to face throughout the dressing process. (See also page 1.)

## Timing

The rate at which the carer gives instructions is very important. Instructions given too quickly may confuse the learner; if given too slowly their meaning may be unclear and the learner's concentration lost. The teacher/carer must find the correct balance for each individual. Time must always be allowed for one instruction to be understood, and a response made, before that instruction is repeated or a second instruction is given. (See also page 4.)

## Language

Before teaching can begin the teacher must gain the learner's attention. Eye contact should be maintained when speaking and when using visual cues. The teacher may need to turn the learner's face to look towards her. When communicating with a learner who finds eye contact difficult to maintain, a compromise may be necessary (see page 46). Instructions should be short, using a limited, consistent vocabulary, and, if necessary, they should be repeated. The level of language used should be reduced until there is some understanding. Vocabulary and sentence length should be built up slowly. If there is more than one carer/teacher, they must all use the same vocabulary at the same level.

## Signing

Visual information remains in the memory longer than information that is heard. For this reason, visual cues are valuable for teaching any skill. Visual cues are a part of communication and should always be used as well as speech, not as a substitute. Different visual cues will suit different people's needs, eg simple mimes of activities while giving instructions, pointing to garments whilst naming them, pointing to different parts of the body and indicating which garments should go where, or formalised systems of signing (eg Makaton). Makaton is a language programme which uses signs in a very structured way, accompanying normal grammatical speech. It is used by many people and can be learnt by attending short workshops that are held all over the country (details of courses and your local Makaton representative can be obtained from the Makaton Vocabulary Development Project, see Appendix II). Once a successful method of communication has been discovered, all carers should use it.

## Symbols and pictures

Some people find it useful to follow pictorial sequences (photographs, diagrams or symbols, mounted in books, wall charts or on flash cards) to help them to understand or remember different aspects of the dressing process. These symbols should again be used as a supplement not as a replacement for speech. As with other forms of guidance, visual and verbal instructions should be gradually withdrawn as the task is learnt.

## Recording progress

Alongside the records of mastered dressing skills, the carer must record useful visual cues (ie signs, symbols or pictures), and what vocabulary has been used. Progress and change in those areas must also be recorded so that a consistent level of communication is maintained. (See also page 14.)

## Summary

- An assessment is important to find the nature of each person's communication difficulties.

- Visual and auditory distractions should be excluded.

- Face-to-face teaching is important.

- Consider the learner's rate of understanding and response when giving instructions.

- The teacher must be prepared to try all forms of communication to make herself understood.

- When a level of effective communication has been found it should be used consistently and records kept.

- Signing, miming and symbols should be used *with* the spoken word.

## LIMITED HEARING AND VISION

See also Visual impairment on page 26.

### The learner

Touch on its own, without sight or hearing, is not an efficient method of receiving or storing information; learning will therefore take longer when the learner is visually and hearing impaired. The learner will not have the chance to learn by observing, may not recognise the need for, or the result of, different activities, and may not be motivated to repeat the activity.

### The teacher

When caring for a person who has a dual sensory impairment, it is wise to keep the number of people who interact with him to the minimum. When learning skills, he should be taught to recognise the teacher by some consistent, identifiable feature. Having a small number of familiar carers will help the learner to understand what to expect from each person and what they expect from him. A consistent approach from his group of carers will give the learner security to experiment with new skills.

In residential units a small group of staff could be identified as keyworkers, so that there is at least one familiar person on duty during each shift. When staff levels are low volunteers could be recruited to keep a small group of carers involved with each visually and hearing impaired person. (See also page 2.)

## Environment

A person with a hearing and visual impairment uses his hands to receive tactile information, but may hear and see little that encourages him to explore the environment beyond the reach of his arms. The carer needs to encourage him to explore the environment and use his body, so that he can participate in any activity. The carer must take each person through all the movements necessary to make him realise the flexibility of his body and to enable him to explore and interpret the environment so that he becomes involved in self-care skills.

For those with limited hearing and vision who are learning to understand their environment and routine, boundaries are important. When learning dressing skills, each session should always take place in the same room with furniture and fittings arranged in exactly the same way. A familiar environment will give the learner a greater security and encourage him to use his initiative when carrying out tasks and learning new skills. (See also pages 1 and 29.)

## Timing/routine

Time boundaries are essential for establishing a routine for getting dressed and undressed. Since people with a dual impairment have no way of knowing what is to happen next, carers must establish a pattern so that they know what to expect in different situations. If the teacher precedes each task with a set routine, the learner can anticipate what is to happen, eg if she washes him before dressing begins.

When teaching skills carers must keep to a set routine so that the learner will become familiar with, and be able to predict, each stage. (See also pages 4 and 30).

## Clothing selection and storage

See pages 26-28.

## Communication/guidance

Each individual will have a different way of communicating, using either formal or informal signs and signals. Once an effective means of

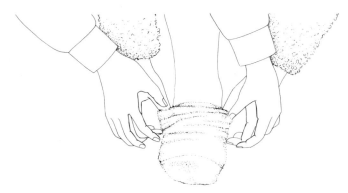

*The teacher guides the learner's hands through the task*

communicating has been established, the signs and signals used must be monitored and recorded so that all carers use them consistently. Two-way communication is important to ensure that the learner and teacher have the same understanding of what the task is, and what is expected of each of them. The carer must find a way of communicating to help the learner anticipate what is about to happen, eg touching the sole of his foot before putting a sock on, touching the top of his head gently before putting a jersey on, gently tugging the lapel of his dressing gown before removing it.

The teacher should make use of any residual vision or hearing – by trying to maintain close eye contact while communicating; by using speech to reinforce all signals; or by speaking close to the learner's ear.

The teacher can pass on information through her hands in a 'hands-on' or 'co-active' movement. The teacher positions herself behind the learner who sits on the floor, on her lap or on a stool or low backed chair without arms. This position allows her to guide the learner's hands through the task with his arms and the rest of his body at a natural angle for the activity. This method of guidance can be used initially to help the learner to explore the environment and his own body, and later to feel and recognise different garments and learn how and where they go on his body. When the teacher feels that the learner is anticipating what is going to happen next in dressing or undressing, physical guidance can be reduced and the learner will gradually be able to carry out the task independently. A teacher may only be able to receive messages from the learner through careful observation, and she must be aware of, and respond to, any changes.

## Recording

Because uniformity and consistency are necessary, records that are simple to follow, regularly updated and easily accessible, are vital to keep all carers in touch with each individual's needs. Environment, timing, communication and incentives should all be recorded together with progress in dressing skills. (See also page 14.)

## Discrimination skills

See pages 16-21.

## Teaching methods

If the learner is guided through the actions needed to get dressed and undressed, the tasks will slowly become more familiar to him. The teacher must gradually withdraw physical assistance as the learner completes tasks unaided. The task will have been taught in a familiar environment with a consistent approach from the teacher, who follows a set routine. When the whole task can be completed unaided and the learner understands how and why it must be done, the teacher can introduce some variety into the routine, so that the learner can adapt his skills. Alterations can start gradually, but the aim is to make the skill part of everyday life, so that the learner can dress or undress at appropriate times of day and in different places, eg at the swimming pool. Accepting new elements in a familiar routine is difficult; the teacher must be certain that the time for changes is right, and offer the learner support while these are introduced and accepted. (See also pages 6-12.)

## Incentives

The learner with an auditory and visual impairment is not able to see or hear the results of his hard work, so it is important to find some way of motivating him to continue learning. His attention should be drawn to the results of getting dressed or undressed, eg dressing to keep warm, dressing to get involved in activities, dressing to have breakfast, undressing to get into bed. He is unlikely to be motivated by praise or smiles, so the teacher must find an appropriate incentive for each learner (see pages 12-14).

Success is important when learning a new skill; it will give the learner the confidence to try other tasks.

## Other activities

See Appendix I and page 31.

## *Summary*

- Learning will take longer if touch is the only method of receiving information.

- Any residual hearing and vision should be utilised.

- The number of people involved in teaching a person who has a dual sensory impairment should be kept to a minimum.

- Consistency is important in the environment, approaches to teaching and methods of communication and guidance.

- Setting boundaries to precede different tasks and following a definite routine are important to help the learner predict what will happen next.

- Variations in routine and environment can be introduced gradually when basic skills have become familiar and the learner has succeeded consistently.


# DIFFICULTIES WITH ATTENTION AND CONCENTRATION

People with severe and profound learning difficulties may never be able to dress completely independently, but it is still important that maximum participation is encouraged. This may be achieved through increased attention and concentration on the task and a further awareness of why and how it takes place. Careful thought should be given to each person's abilities and needs so that the best method of encouraging increased involvement can be found.


## Timing

It may take a long time before each skill is understood and mastered, but teaching time may need to be limited because the learner's attention span is short. (See also page 4.)


## Teaching

The teacher may have to start by stimulating the learner to take an interest and watch the dressing process. This passive participation may have to continue for some time until the learner begins to be more aware of himself, the need to get dressed and the different processes that must be carried out in order to get dressed. Incentives may be needed to encourage this initial attention and concentration on what is happening (see pages 12-14). The

*Example VIII: Encouraging participation when getting dressed.*

| | Name | | | |
|---|---|---|---|---|
| | Date | | | |
| 1. | Sits on bed when it is time to get dressed. | I | | |
| 2. | Makes eye contact. | V | | |
| 3. | Looks at each garment before it is put on. | V | | |
| 4. | Lifts arms for 'T' shirt to be put on. | V G ∗ | | |
| 5. | Lifts feet for pants/socks trousers/shoes to be put on. | P∗ | | |
| 6. | Stands up for trousers/ pants to be pulled on. | P∗ | | |

I = Independent
V = Verbal instructions
G = Gestured instructions
P = Physical help
∗ = Reward given (praise and smile)

learner's attention to the task may be attracted if the teacher gives assistance during dressing from the front, although the teacher's face may then prove to be more interesting to the learner than the task! If this is the case then assistance given from the side may help the learner to concentrate on the dressing process. In example VIII (see above), the man is being encouraged to notice what is happening and to begin to participate in dressing; the carer is not expecting him to be actively involved in putting on garments at this stage.

The teacher may eventually offer incentives to encourage more active participation, teaching the skills needed to get dressed step-by-step. As

*Example IX: Encouraging skills when getting dressed and undressed*

| Name | | | | |
|---|---|---|---|---|
| Date | 12-11 | 19-11 | 26-11 | 3-12 |
| Grips bottom edge of 'T' shirt. | V.<br>P | V.<br>P | V<br>P | V<br>P |
| Pulls 'T' shirt up to under arms. | P | P | P | P |
| Removes arms from sleeve. | P | P | P | P |
| Pulls 'T' shirt from neck to chin. | P | P | P | P |
| Pulls 'T' shirt from chin to top of head. | V<br>P | V G<br>P | V G<br>P | V<br>G * |
| Pulls 'T' shirt off from top of head | V<br>* | V<br>* | I * | I * |

I = Independent
G = Gestured instructions
P = Physical help
V = Verbal instructions
* = Reward given (praise and smile)

mentioned in Chapter 1 (see page 8), it is wise to build on existing skills. People who have difficulty in understanding the task may have some natural physical responses that can be used to encourage the development of dressing skills, eg a man who pulls coverings away from his face can be encouraged to removed a 'T' shirt from his head (see example IX above).

## Extra activities to improve dressing skills

People with severe learning difficulties and problems with concentration, understanding and attention can improve their skills each time that clothing is put on or taken off (see page 4). At other times during the day, skills associated with dressing can be practised when there may be more time for exploration and experiments. All activities should be appropriate to each person's age and ability (see Appendix I).

## Summary

- The learner may need to be stimulated to improve his concentration and attention span before learning dressing skills.

- Existing skills or responses can be used to encourage dressing skills.

- Extra activities throughout the day can be made use of to reinforce self-awareness and dressing skills and an understanding of body parts and clothing and footwear.


# PERCEPTUAL PROBLEMS

Those whose conditions have resulted in abnormalities in the make-up of the brain, may have resulting difficulties in interpreting and understanding what they see, touch and hear. This is a problem of perception. Dressing demands co-ordination of the hand and arm and a recognition and awareness of all parts of the body: someone learning to dress must be able to recognise where his body is in relation to other objects in the room, be able to discriminate clothing from other objects in the room, recognise where and how a garment goes on his body and be aware of all areas in his field of vision. A perceptual disorder could interfere with the abilities described and could be the cause of a child or adult's failure to learn dressing skills.

If there are problems with perception, help should be sought from a psychologist, occupational therapist, nurse or teacher so that methods of compensating for, or overcoming, these problems can be taught before work begins on the more complex task of dressing.


## Selection of clothes

A person who has problems with perception will find it easier when first learning dressing skills if clothes have a clearly defined front, back, inside, outside, top and bottom, have simple fasteners and are easy to put on and take off (see page 57). Garments with visual and tactile clues will also make it easier to position clothes on the body.


## Storage of clothes

A person who finds it difficult to recognise and discriminate between different garments needs a well organised storage system for clothing (see pages 89-92).

## Environment

Perceptual problems may result in visual problems or lack of awareness of parts or one side of the body. If this is the case, the teacher should organise the environment so that all approaches can be made from the side or area that the learner tends to neglect. Clothing should be stored or handed to the learner from his neglected side, so that he gets into the habit of looking or turning in that direction. (See also page 1.)

## Timing

Establishing a routine that can be followed every time dressing and undressing is practised may help the learner to compensate for perceptual problems. The teacher should consider each person's ability and concentrate on each task in turn rather than on the whole dressing process. Plenty of time should be allocated for regular practising. (See also page 4.)

## Learner and teacher

An occupational therapist or psychologist may be able to carry out a formal assessment of the learner's perceptual loss, but the carer should be aware of how these problems affect each person's ability to learn dressing skills and adapt her teaching methods accordingly. (See also pages 2-3.)

## Teaching methods

The carer should use a consistent vocabulary, together with gestures and physical clues when appropriate, and the clothes should, at first, be set out in the same place, ready to put on, each day. Any physical guidance used to help those with poor co-ordination should be from behind so that the learner can see how the movements take place and feel their arms move in relation to the rest of their body (people who have increased muscle tone should be guided from the front as guidance from the back tends to encourage them to push backwards, which interferes with function). Mirrors can be used to aid dressing, but may be confusing for those who have difficulty identifying the different sides of their body. The learner should be encouraged to look down at his body when dressing and use the mirror to look at the overall effect when fully dressed. (See also pages 6-12.)

## Extra activities to improve dressing skills

See Appendix I.

## Body awareness

The learner must be aware of his body's shape and how it moves, and also understand how clothing goes on his body before he can learn to get dressed. Advice on how to improve a person's concept of his body can be sought from occupational therapists, physiotherapists and teachers. Massage, rubbing and touching will help to make people aware of the different parts of their body. Activities that involve guiding a person to move in different ways will help him to understand how his limbs can move independently and in relation to each other. By touch and physical contact with other people through exercises, a person with perceptual problems will learn how other people's bodies move and may be able to relate it to his own. Increased knowledge of his own body, its range of movement and limitations in the environment will help to improve his self-help skills.

## *Summary*

- Consistency is important in routine, vocabulary and environment.

- Clothes and footwear with visual and tactile clues may be an advantage.

- The ability to discriminate between garments will be helped by organised clothing and footwear storage.

- Carers should find out how perceptual problems are affecting dressing skills and encourage the learner to use other skills to compensate.

- Extra activities can be undertaken to improve self awareness and specific dressing skills.

## LACK OF CO-OPERATION

A carer who encounters someone who refuses to co-operate in dressing should try to discover and then remove the underlying reason. Some people may so dislike the clothes chosen for them, perhaps because the fabric or style is uncomfortable, that they are reluctant to get dressed. Allowing people to choose and buy their own clothes will ensure that colour, style and feel are acceptable. The carer should offer clothes in a wide choice of fabrics and styles and make sure that the wearer tries them on when shopping.

If someone is particularly fond of one outfit and refuses to dress in any other, the carer should involve the learner in the washing of these clothes to try and make it clear to him that, while they are being washed, he will have to wear something else. When shopping, the carer should point out similar clothes that may be equally attractive to him. (See page 52, inappropriate styles, and page 20, discrimination between clean and dirty clothes.)

## Timing

Some people may be reluctant to become actively involved with dressing because they prefer to dress at a particular time. They may prefer to stay in bed longer in the morning and sacrifice a long breakfast so that they can dress when they feel more awake; or to get up and have breakfast in their dressing gown and slippers, dressing after breakfast when they feel more alert and nourished. If this routine does not fit in with that of the rest of the household, the carer should find another, more acceptable, time when the learner is prepared to learn dressing skills, eg when undressing at night, or when changing for sports. The carer should continue to give assistance in the morning, when time and motivation are in short supply, but once dressing skills have been mastered the learner should be encouraged to help in the mornings as well. (See also page 4.)

## Environment

The learner may dislike the environment in which he is expected to get dressed and undressed – it may be too public, too isolated, too cold, too hot; he may prefer to get dressed in the bathroom or bedroom, or with the curtains closed and the light on or *vice versa*; or he may prefer to stand or sit on the bed, chair or floor. While carers will be reluctant to disrupt the routine of the whole household to accommodate the needs of one person, they may want to introduce simple changes in the dressing environment to see if they increase a learner's motivation. (See also page 1.)

## Teacher

The learner will respond differently to different teachers; consideration should therefore be given as to who is the best person to teach dressing skills. She should have the ability to encourage maximum participation so that the learner improves his skills and enjoys the increased independence that results from learning to dress himself. (See also page 2.)

## Learner

Carers should find out why the learner is reluctant to acquire independent dressing skills. The learner may like the attention he gets when he is dressed by a particular carer and be reluctant to lose this attention. The carer could remedy this situation by giving the learner more attention when he is actively participating in dressing than when he is not. Increased co-operation may be encouraged if the learner is taught why he should get dressed and what opportunities are open to him when he is dressed – going out to shop, for instance. (See also page 3.)

## Teaching methods

The learner may be reluctant to co-operate because he dislikes the methods of guidance used. Some people do not like physical contact or being face to face with someone who is giving them instructions. The teacher could seek a more relaxed approach for that individual – guiding him by words and gestures rather than by physical contact, by sitting next to him while he is dressing to reduce the amount of face to face contact, or by leaving the room (or occupying herself in another part of it) from time to time so that the learner has a chance to experiment without being watched. Spoken demands may also lead to reluctance to co-operate, especially if the learner has limited understanding of speech. Teachers should look at alternative methods of guidance or slow down their rate of speech (see page 32). (See also pages 7-12).

The incentives offered may not appeal sufficiently to that particular learner, and alternatives should be sought (see pages 12-14).

## Other activities to increase dressing skills

Any other activity involving getting dressed and undressed in different situations, especially if there is no pressure to succeed and mistakes can be made, will help the carer to assess the learner's existing skills and may give her some insight into why he does not co-operate when learning dressing skills (see Appendix I).

## *Summary*

● Carers should try to discover the reasons why the learner will not co-operate.

● The cause could be due to: clothing, timing, environment, teacher, teaching approach or lack of motivation.

● Every effort should be made to overcome the cause without disrupting the rest of the household.

• Every opportunity should be taken to introduce the skills needed for dressing in other activities undertaken during the day.


## FURTHER READING

Ruston, R. *Dressing for disabled people: a manual for nurses and others.* London, Disabled Living Foundation, 1977, revised 1982.

(an illustrated guide to methods of dressing and undressing for people with physical limitations)

Dunn, M L. *Pre-dressing skills: skill starters for self-help development.* Arizona, Communication Skill Builders, 1983 (Distributed by Winslow Press)

(a workbook for nurses, teachers and therapists to guide them in teaching dressing to developmentally delayed and physically handicapped children)

Finnie, N. *Handling the young cerebral palsied child at home.* London, Heinemann, 1968, revised 1974, reprint 1981.

(discusses causes and solutions to problems related to muscle tone disorders in children and looks at ways maximum independence can be encouraged)

Golding, R and Goldsmith, L. *The caring persons guide to handling the severely multiply handicapped.* London, Macmillan, 1986.

(a practical manual for all carers aimed at complementing physiotherapists input by ensuring good, 24 hour physical management to maximise function and minimise deformity)

Fullwood, D. *A start to independence for your visually impaired child.* (Australia) Royal Victoria Institute for the Blind, 1986. Available for sale from the National Library for the Handicapped Child.

(a practical guide for parents and direct carers on teaching independence skills to a person who has a visual handicap)

Ellis, D. ed. *Sensory impairments in mentally handicapped people.* London, Croom Helm, 1986.

(Chapter 16 by Tony Best explains how a visual handicap affects the ability to learn, and the most effective method of teaching skills to a person who has a visual handicap)

Freeman, P. *The deaf blind baby: a programme of care*. London, Heinemann, 1985.

(a practical guide for parents and direct carers on how to develop their babies' full potential)

Wyman, R. *Multiply handicapped children*. London, Souvenir Press. 1986.

(first hand experience and advice from parents of children with dual sensory impairments on how to overcome problems encountered)


## Other useful material


*The cerebral palsied child: method of dressing.* 373/1-2
Tape slide presentation *and* video – sale or hire
Available from: Camera Talks Ltd, 197 Botley Road, Oxford OX2 0HE (tel: 0865 726625)

(shows the development of the physical skills necessary to get dressed and the importance of positioning to maximise function)

*Making progress*
Video – sale or hire
Available from: Concord Films, 201 Felixstowe Road, Ipswich, Suffolk IP3 9BJ (tel: 0473 726012)

(shows how a group of people with severe learning difficulties and challenging behaviours were encouraged to develop skills leading towards involvement in functional activities)

*Looking after myself*
Video – sale or hire
Available from: ILEA Consortium, Jack Tizard School, Finlay Street, London SW6 6HB (tel: 01 736 8877)

(six short programmes aimed at teenagers with learning difficulties to encourage an interest and participation in self care skills)

# 3

# Selecting clothes

First impressions make a strong impact. It is therefore important, particularly as people become increasingly aware of the need to integrate those with learning difficulties into the community, that someone with such difficulties should have the same chance as everyone else to make a good first impression. For this reason, clothing assumes a particular significance.

People with learning difficulties have the right to choose and buy their own clothes and also to choose what to wear each day. However, some may choose to dress in a style that may lead other members of the public to have a prejudiced or biased opinion about their behaviour or personality and so prevent their full integration and acceptance. Carers should protect each person's right to choose; this chapter investigates ways in which someone with learning difficulties can be encouraged to choose clothes from a wide range of styles to suit his tastes and needs and to express his individuality in a way that does not isolate him from the rest of the community.

## ENCOURAGING CHOICE

Choice is difficult for those who have never before been faced with it. But since it is by exercising choice that all of us can have some control over our lives, it is important that even those who are initially reluctant should be encouraged to make choices so that they too can enjoy the satisfaction of making their own decisions, however small.

### Ways of encouraging choice

1. The best way of communicating with each individual must be found to discover what he likes and dislikes.
2. Discussion about styles – eg what suits a particular person's figure or age, what colours accentuate his good points and detract from problem areas – would help those who can understand the concept.

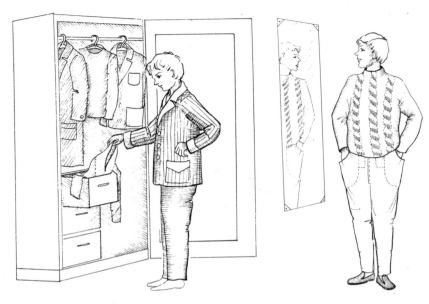

*Choosing from the wardrobe*          *Self appraisal in the mirror*

3. Carers should encourage an interest in colours and clothes, and point out to learners what people whom they see around them, on television, in books and when window shopping, are wearing.

4. Learners could be encouraged to take an interest in the feel and colour of the different fabrics so that they can discriminate between what is appealing and what is not.

5. Plenty of time must be allowed for choices to be made.

6. Initially, the learner should be asked to choose between two garments from the wardrobe; as his confidence grows, the selection can be gradually increased.

7. Feedback about how each chosen outfit looks, what colours and styles suit each person, is valuable.

8. Self appraisal in the mirror should be encouraged to increase self awareness and interest in appearance.

9. Each individual's choices and decisions about other activities during the day should be encouraged and respected. Once a person has more control over how he wants to spend his time, then he or his carer will have more idea about what clothes will suit that life style.

## When choosing what to wear each day

Some carers may find that encouraging independent choice each morning is too time consuming. Altering the daily or weekly routine or limiting the choices available may be a way of overcoming this problem.

1. Each person could be given time to select a complete outfit at bed time, and lay it out ready to put on the next day.

2. One or two mornings a week could be devoted to choosing clothes and giving feedback about choices that have been made (eg when more carers are available, when other residents or family members are not at home or not requiring supervision).

3. The wearer could be offered a carefully limited choice, eg between two complete outfits, choosing the colour or which pair of trousers or jumper he wants to wear, while the carer selects other clothes to match these choices.

Methods of encouraging and learning about choice (see page 49) need not be practised in the mornings or evenings during dressing and undressing but can be practised at any time with direct carers in the home or with teachers, instructors and friends in the course of daily activities.

## When guidance is needed

### When mistakes are made

Everyone likes to wear clothes that are comfortable and make them feel self confident. The mistakes made in choosing clothes are usually communicated to the wearer through other people's reactions or because he feels uncomfortable. People with learning difficulties should not be protected from this valuable feedback. Carers should allow experimentation and expect some mistakes to occur; they must make it clear to the person making the choice how he looks, *why* he looks 'good' or 'not so good', or let him discover for himself how uncomfortable or impractical a certain style may be.

### Communication difficulties

Everyone can respond to choice and it is very important that people with severe learning difficulties, who may not be able to communicate their needs, still have their likes and dislikes taken into account when choosing clothes. By observing people's reactions in many different situations, carers should be able to discover their preferences, eg what colours each

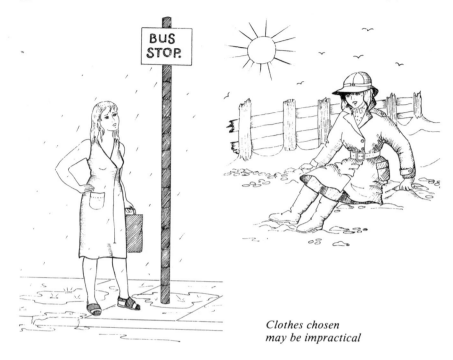

*Clothes chosen
may be impractical*

person prefers, what styles he finds most comfortable and what fabrics he likes to feel next to his skin.

## Inappropriate styles

Those who choose to dress in an inappropriate style that draws attention to their disabilities rather than their attributes, should receive some guidance. Carers should make sure that they have access to a wide range of styles that are currently available so that they can select the type of clothes they prefer. Encouraging people to be aware of different styles and to learn how they look to others should be included in their general education.

## Age-appropriate clothing

If an individual dresses in clothing that is inappropriate for his age, some people immediately jump to the conclusion that he is attached to the local hospital or hostel. It is therefore important in this situation that carers should try to guide the learner's choice towards clothes appropriate to his age; carers of the same sex and similar age can often be seen by him as role models, although a carer should never try to impose her style onto others. Mixing with people of a similar age in many different situations may give the learner some insight into what styles are popular, and shopping in stores or departments that cater for his age group will make him realise the wide range of styles that are available and appropriate. (See Chapter 1 for teaching discrimination skills, pages 16-21.)

## When choosing clothes for someone else

Choice is subjective, and if the carer has no alternative but to choose clothes for the learner, she should try not to impose her style, culture, taste or standards on him. Parents and carers who have a close relationship with the learner will have some insight into the type of clothes that suit his life-style and age.

When there is more than one carer, they should all discuss the learner's needs and, if necessary, decide to guide his choice of dress so that it is more appropriate. This decision should not be taken lightly and should be open to review if, or when, that person gains more insight into how he looks and is able to take more responsibility for his choice of clothing. Alternatively, one carer who is familiar with the learner's needs, life style, culture and preferences, may be chosen by the staff group to speak for him. Some establishments ask an external committee or individual to decide who should speak for each person.

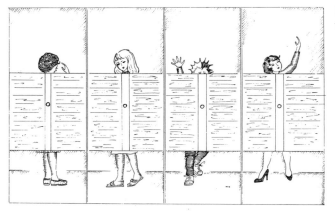

*Visiting shops is a valuable activity.*

# SHOPPING

When choosing clothes in a shop those who are not used to making choices will find it easier at first if the number of garments is limited and they are given plenty of time to look, feel and try on the garments, while they decide what they want. As they gain more confidence in decision-making the range should be extended. Visiting shops is a valuable activity, not only because it gives people the opportunity to choose clothes from a wide range of styles but also because it allows them to practise social skills and to come into contact with a wide range of people.

In residential units it is often helpful to keep a written record of what clothes each person has, what his needs are, what styles, fabric and shops he prefers, any cultural or religious clothing specifications and any guidance he may require when making choices. This record should be kept by a key worker or a member of the care staff who has taken responsibility for clothing.

Everyone should have the opportunity to go shopping in the community for their own clothes, but some carers may find it difficult to arrange this because of lack of time, transport difficulties or because of poor toilet or access facilities in shopping centres. These problems can often be overcome by investigating and calling on resources in the local community.

## Transport

Those who have no transport of their own, have difficulty using public transport or live in an area where public transport is inadequate, can benefit from the wide range of assistance with local journeys that is available. Alternative forms of transport as well as assistance for those

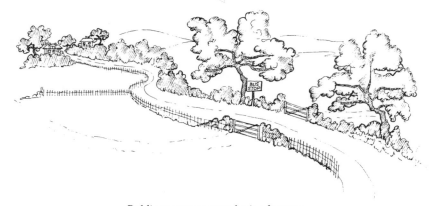

*Public transport may be inadequate*

using public transport can often be arranged. The Citizens Advice Bureaux should have details of local help; alternatively a request to the National Advisory Unit for Community Transport, (accompanied by a stamped addressed envelope) giving specific details of the type of information required, should elicit the necessary information (see Appendix II).

Local voluntary organisations, about which the nearest Citizens Advice Bureau should have details, often provide door-to-door transport in minibuses or private cars.

The Department of Transport publishes a guide, *Door to Door*, available from local authorities or transport operators, which includes details of the practical and financial assistance available to those who have difficulty using public transport.

## Local shops

Shop managers can be approached for information on the availability of lifts and toilets and will often allow customers with mobility problems to use the service lift if no customer lift is available. Managers can give advice on their shops' refund and exchange policies; these allow shoppers to take a selection of garments home to try on when there is more space and time for decisions to be made. Managers can advise on quiet times during the week when the staff will have more time to help; some shops have late-night shopping facilities.

## Community team

Most districts now have a community team – run by social services or the health service and made up of psychiatrists, social workers, community nurses, psychologists, occupational therapists, speech therapists, physiotherapists and assistants – who work with families and people who have learning difficulties. Most teams can be contacted through health centres or by telephoning their office directly (the number should be available from the general hospital or social service office). Increasing people's independence when using shops and public transport is an area in which the community team offers its expertise. The team may also provide contacts with other local agencies who can offer assistance, eg a 'sitting' service, providing staff (vetted by the community team) who can sometimes be used to care for other children in a family, leaving parents more time to shop or choose clothes with the child who has a learning difficulty.

## Help from voluntary bodies

The nearest library or Citizens Advice Bureau will give information on local voluntary bodies and organisations. The Volunteer Centre UK will, on receipt of a stamped addressed envelope, identify the nearest volunteer bureau. The teams of volunteers from the 350 volunteer bureaux throughout the country will provide a variety of services, depending on the area and resources, such as help with transport to and from the shops and assistance in the shops.

Local Womens Royal Voluntary Service (WRVS) offices are listed in the telephone directory and they welcome requests for help with shopping. The type of assistance they can offer will depend on the resources of the local branch. Specialist bodies, such as One to One and Advocacy Alliance, have been set up in some areas; they can provide 'advocates' to accompany people on shopping trips, offering whatever type or level of guidance is needed (see Appendix II for addresses).

## CLOTHES FOR EASY DRESSING

When first assisting with dressing or when teaching dressing skills, the carer should try to provide a choice of clothes that will make the process quick and easy. However, a person who has learnt the basic dressing skills should not have his choice limited in this way.

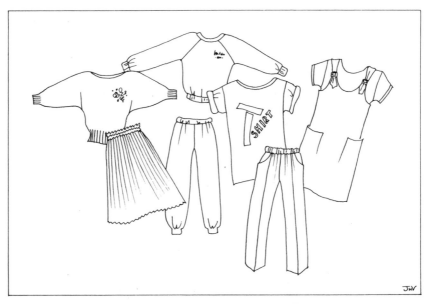

*A choice of clothes for easy dressing*

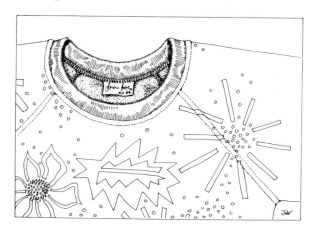

*Textures and patterns help to identify a garment's inside, outside, back and front*

## Styles

The number of clothes worn should, where possible, be kept to a minimum. Styles should be simple and loose fitting or have some 'give'. Clothes with large openings, loose fitting armholes or raglan sleeves will make the process of putting on and taking off easier. A clearly defined front and back, inside and outside, will make it easier to position clothes on the body, eg fasteners or labels in the same position on each garment, patterns, prints or other features on the front, well defined seams or different textures inside and outside.

## Fabrics

Garments made of fabrics that stretch are usually easy to put on and take off. Those made of rigid fabrics can be lined with a smooth silky cloth to make dressing and undressing easier. When encouraging a person to dress or to co-operate during assisted dressing, the carer might find it helpful if the learner wears fabrics that feel 'good' against his skin.

## Fasteners

To make dressing easier, fasteners should be kept to a minimum; indeed elasticated styles that have *no* fasteners may be ideal for those who need assistance to get dressed and those who are learning the first skills needed to dress independently. The number of styles without fasteners is, however, limited.

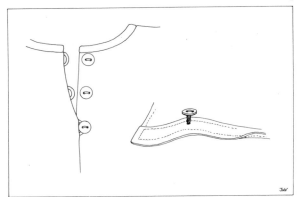

*Looped button holes
and buttons with a long
shank*

The position of fasteners is important. They should be easy to reach and not likely to cause discomfort to the wearer; the front mid-line position is usually the best.

The wearer's physical ability and learning potential should be considered when choosing fasteners to make sure that he can manipulate the fasteners independently or with minimal assistance.

## Buttons

Small buttons are often difficult both to do up and undo; smooth, flat, hard buttons of 2cm or more in diameter with a slightly raised rim are usually the easiest to manage, although some people prefer toggles to buttons. If buttons are sewn on with a long shank or with elastic thread they are usually easier to manage. Looped button holes of fabric or elastic can be a satisfactory substitute for those who cannot manage slit button holes, while vertical button holes and those that are slightly larger than the button make dressing easier – although, if the buttons are in a position where they will be subjected to strain, they may come undone.

## Zips

Zip fasteners are generally quicker and easier to do up than buttons, and garments can be bought with various weights and styles of zip. Nylon zips are less conspicuous and less likely to 'catch' the skin or other garments than metal ones, but they are not as strong (eg in trousers or jeans). Open-ended zips make access easier but are more difficult to align and fasten together than closed-end zips. Tags, such as rings, tassels, loops of

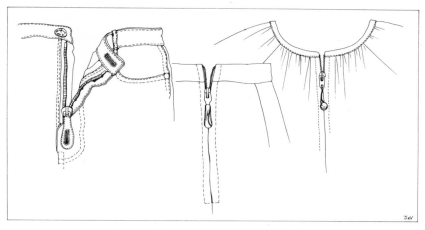

*Fabric, ribbon and beads added to zip tags*

fabric, can be added easily and discreetly to zip tags so that those who have difficulty manipulating conventional tags find them easier to fasten. Loops can also be added to the base of a closed-end zip so that it can be anchored with one finger when the zip is being closed, and to both sides of an open ended zip so that they are easier to grasp when the ends are being locked together.

## Hooks and eyes

Small hooks and eyes are difficult to see, feel and manipulate. They could be replaced with corset or trouser hooks if these do not spoil the look of the garment. On heavier garments, large sew-on trouser hooks and bars may be easier to manipulate than those fixed through the fabric of ready-made garments.

## Press fasteners

These come in a variety of sizes and can be sewn on or riveted. Those with a button sewn over the top or the riveted type with a button backing are easier to manipulate than the conventional sew-in variety. Poppers may not be strong enough in areas where there is tension (eg the waistband).

## Velcro

This touch and close fastener, which consists of hooked and looped surfaces that lock together on contact and can be ripped apart again, can be managed by those with very limited use of their upper limbs. To prevent discomfort, the hooked section should always be sewn on so that it faces away from the skin. Velcro should be sewn on in small sections (2cm is usually sufficient), because long strips can distort fine fabric and are difficult to align (4cm lengths are the maximum that should be used). Small dots of velcro may not be strong enough for any area where there is strain. When washing, velcro must always be closed – so that it cannot catch on other parts of the garment and so that the hooked section does not become 'furred'.

Velcro can be a hindrance when dressing as the hooked surface tends to snag other garments. In addition, some children and adults who enjoy the sound and feel of velcro tend to play continuously with the fastener and eventually cause the clothes to gape, and people who are used to velcro have a tendency to apply the opening technique (pulling) to other fasteners.

Velcro is undoubtably valuable for those with limited hand function, but it must not be seen as the answer to all fastening problems.

People with learning difficulties who understand how to fasten velcro are just as likely to be able to manipulate other conventional fasteners if the task is broken down into manageable steps. Anyone with the physical abilities required to manipulate conventional fasteners should be encouraged to do so to increase the range of clothing available to them.

## FOOTWEAR

Consideration should be given to each individual's needs as well as his preferences when selecting footwear. The shoe should be well fitting to maintain foot health and be made in a style that is attractive to the wearer. A well fitting shoe should be long enough and deep enough for the foot (allowing 1cm between the end of the longest toe and the inside front of the shoe), with a firm fastening around the instep holding the heel into the back of the shoe. Without this firm fastening, the foot will slide forward, and the resulting impaction could lead to curled toes. Fashion shoes rarely combine all these points and adults should be encouraged to wear fashion shoes only for special occasions and for short periods of time. Children whose feet are still developing should always wear well fitting shoes as any constriction or imbalance might lead to permanent deformity or problems with walking.

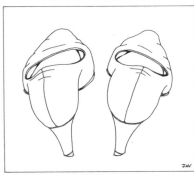

*Worn heels cause imbalance*

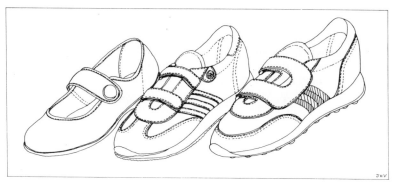

*Easy shoe fasteners*

Since high heeled shoes will push the foot forward, anyone choosing to wear them should be advised to look for a style with a firm fastener at the instep to prevent crushed toes. High heels must be checked for wear at the edges; this is usually more marked than on the heels of flat shoes, and will alter the base when walking.

## Shoe fasteners

Those who have difficulty manipulating fasteners can wear slip-on shoes as long as they bear in mind that, as such shoes tend to fall off while walking, the toes will curl up to hold the shoes on, and possibly cause toe deformities. The carer should ensure that the front of slip-on shoes extends high enough up the instep to prevent the shoe falling off. Elastic gussets may serve this purpose but the hold must be firm enough to keep the heel in place.

Laces are a common shoe fastener and give good support at the instep. Many people find it difficult to tie shoe laces but they can sometimes be successfully replaced by elastic laces which are left permanently tied, converting the shoe into a slip-on (the tongue may need a stitch at one side to prevent it slipping down). Those who are unable to dress independently should choose shoes with a large opening so that foot comfort can be checked. Lace-ups in a Derby or Gibson style open wide to give easy access to the foot when the laces are undone (see pages 76-77).

Buckles can provide a firm hold on a bar across the instep but, if small, may be difficult to fasten and unfasten. Press studs can sometimes be placed under them for those who find this fastener difficult.

Velcro, which is becoming quite a common shoe fastener, is easy to do up and undo. It can provide a firm hold if kept free from dust and fluff with a stiff toothbrush and left closed when the shoe is not being worn.

## Materials

Leather is the preferable material for shoe uppers as it allows perspiration to escape and will mould itself in time to accommodate the foot's irregularities; if there is a lining, it must also be of leather if the shoe is to have these properties.

Shoes with synthetic uppers and lining are often cheaper but, since they do not stretch like leather, they must fit perfectly when purchased. The synthetic material will not allow perspiration to pass through.

Shoes with fabric uppers are available and these can be comfortable for some occasions. Training shoes are made in a variety of styles and materials and have become universally popular.

Shoe soles, unlike uppers, are often more suitable if made of synthetic materials as they can be more durable, waterproof, flexible and lighter than traditional leather soles. Soft or cellular materials will give the sole of a shoe more resistance to slipping, as will soles with textured patterns or ridges.

## SELECTING 'SAFE' CLOTHES

Hospitals and residential units, bearing in mind fire hazards, may restrict the type of clothing worn, and carers in the community may also be concerned about a garment's fire resistance. Some fabrics do have flame retardant properties and up-to-date details of these can be obtained from the Clothing Adviser at the Disabled Living Foundation. Supplies officers will be able to give any fabric specifications for their area. The wearer's choice of clothes will be limited if he has to select only those made with flame retardant fabrics.

The risk of being burnt in a clothing-related fire depends not only on the fabric and the garment but also on the environment and the ability of the wearer to sense or react to fire. All these factors must be taken into account when the need for flame retardant fabric is considered.

*Summary*

● Everyone has the right to choose his own clothes, and the style of dress to suit his own culture and life-style.

● Careful guidance may be needed so that each person can learn what is available to suit his age, figure and chosen style of dress.

● When shopping for, or selecting, clothes, local community resources may solve difficulties caused by lack of time or transport.

● Styles and fasteners can be selected to make dressing easier but once someone has learnt the basic dressing skills he should not be limited by these factors when choosing clothes.

● Careful selection of footwear can produce a balance between style, comfort and ease of dressing while maintaining foot health.

● Flammability of garments may be a consideration when selecting clothes.

## FURTHER READING

*Door to door: a guide to transport for disabled people*, 2nd ed. Department of Transport, 1986. Available free of charge from: Door to Door Guide, Freepost, Victoria Road, South Ruislip, Middlesex HA4 0NZ.

**Other useful material**

*Lifestyles.* Training games based on normalisation, Pack 1: Mental Handicap.
Available for sale from: Escata, 6 Pavilion Parade, Brighton, East Sussex BN2 1RA (tel: 0273 695339)

(a study pack for staff involved with day care or residential services for people with learning difficulties. Helps people in the group to examine their own attitudes and values and look at how they can increase opportunities for choice and individuality for people with learning difficulties)

*We can change the future.* London, National Bureau for Handicapped Students, 1986.
Available from: The National Bureau for Handicapped Students, 336 Brixton Road, London SW9 7AA (tel: 01 274 0565)

(a staff training resource comprising a handbook and video designed to teach people about self advocacy, and the rights of people with learning difficulties to speak and make choices for themselves)

# 4

# What affects clothes choice?

Everyone should be given the opportunity to choose their own style of dress from as wide a range of different styles as possible. The wearer's comfort and appearance can be improved if clothes are chosen with care, and this chapter considers how informed selection can overcome specific problems.

## DAMAGE TO CLOTHES AND FOOTWEAR

### Damage due to excessive wear and tear

Clothes subjected to rubbing on callipers, braces or seats, or to excessive wear and tear because of the way in which the wearer moves about (by crawling or sliding on his bottom, for example) will probably wear out very quickly. Carers should first try to discover how this wear and tear can be avoided without restricting freedom of movement. Physiotherapists and occupational therapists could be consulted about padding or smoothing the edges of equipment to prevent rubbing and damage to clothes. Physiotherapists can also assist with mobility problems and may be able to suggest alternatives to crawling and bottom shuffling. A soft floor covering will reduce the amount of wear on the seat, knees or elbows of a garment. If a period of time is set aside each day for the person to move about independently on the floor, he may be willing to wear overalls made of tough fabric (see page 65) over his everyday clothes to give extra protection during that time.

Having considered all methods of avoiding wear and tear, carers should look at the fabric and style of garments to ensure that they will stand up to the extra demands made on them (see pages 65-68).

### Damage caused by inappropriate behaviour

Clothes can be damaged by the wearer who chews, rubs, picks, tears or continually removes them. However, garments that are indestructible or difficult to take off will not necessarily eliminate the problem since such behaviour is often one of the ways in which the wearer conveys messages to carers or other people. If indestructible clothes are worn the wearer may adopt equally destructive behaviour in order to express himself. The carer should try to find out the reason for this behaviour: it could be due to boredom; because the wearer does not have enough to occupy his hands; he may enjoy the sensation and sound of the cloth tearing; the clothing may be uncomfortable; he may not like the colour or style of his clothes; he may have discovered that he attracts more attention than usual after damaging or removing clothes; he may enjoy regular changes of clothes; or he may have found that this behaviour excludes him from an activity he does not enjoy.

A psychologist should be able to help carers to discover the reason for clothing damage and suggest a method of management that will allow the wearer to satisfy his needs through an acceptable activity.

Reinforcing clothes, and using hard wearing fabrics, should only be seen as a temporary measure while the cause of the destructive behaviour is investigated and a solution found.

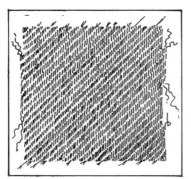

*Denim has a characteristic diagonal stripe.*

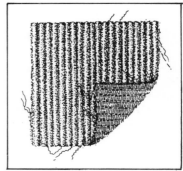

*Check the weave on the underside of a pile fabric*

## Fabric

The durability of fabrics depends on the type of fibres used, how the fibres are spun together to make a yarn, and how the fabric is made up with those yarns. Man-made fibres, like nylon and polyester, are hard wearing but usually feel uncomfortable against the skin. Wool, cotton and other 100% natural fibres do not stand up well to abnormal wear and tear, but a mixture of man-made and natural fibres when spun into a yarn will give durability and comfort, eg polyester/cotton, wool/polyester, wool/nylon, cotton/nylon. The higher the percentage of man-made fibre indicated on the label, the more hard wearing the fabric will be. Any fabric with 2-4%

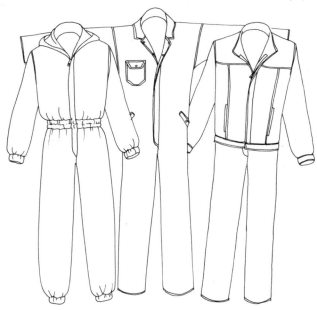

*Strong garments designed for work wear*

elastane fibres (lycra) incorporated in it will wear well because, when strained, the yarns will stretch to some extent instead of breaking. Stretch denim used for jeans has this property; the fabric can often be purchased by the metre to make up into different styles of garment.

Fibres can be spun in different ways to make up the yarns used in fabric manufacture. Plain yarns are tightly spun giving extra strength to the fabric. Fancy yarns with loops or irregular thicknesses are spun more loosely, reducing their strength. Yarns can be woven to make up fabrics, and the closer the weave the stronger the fabric. A close twill weave has a characteristic diagonal line across it, is supple and is one of the hardest wearing fabrics (eg denim). Loosely knitted and woven fabrics do not wear well and are prone to snags, holes and runs. Tightly knitted fabrics, particularly those with a polyester content, are difficult to tear, eg 'T' shirt fabric. Velvet, corduroy and towelling may look thick and strong but all fabrics with a pile finish are only as strong as the base fabric beneath the pile. The under-side of the pile fabric should be checked to see how tightly it is woven.

A 'minimum care finish', indicated on a garment label, although making the fabric easier to wash and iron will reduce its strength.

Smooth surfaced, tightly woven fabrics are advisable for people who tend to pick at loose threads in their clothes. If garments are likely to be chewed or sucked, they should be washed before they are worn for the first time to get rid of excess dye and finishing agents.

## Styles

Garments designed for sport or work are often suitable for everyday use; they are usually stronger and more tear resistant than fashion wear.

## Reinforcements

Points of strain can be reinforced before a garment is worn, to prolong its life and avoid repairs in the future:

- a lining will help to increase a garments strength;
- seams can be reinforced with a second line of stitching; zig-zag or a stretch stitch is advisable when reinforcing a curved seam or stretchy fabric. A strip of tape sewn along the seam line will give extra strength especially on curved seams (eg back seam of trousers);
- vulnerable points in garments can be strengthened with an extra line of stitching or an arrowhead, crowsfoot or bar tack. An extra piece of fabric can be sewn on the under-side of the garment at these points to give extra strength. Areas that often need reinforcement are: the top of pleats, corners of pocket openings, the points on 'V' and square necklines. Garments chosen without these features are not so easily torn;
- buttons that are under strain can be removed and re-stitched with an extra piece of fabric on the under-side; buttons with four holes will be more secure if sewn on with separate threads for each pair of holes; the shank should be long enough to allow the button to be easily manipulated; sewing on buttons with shirring elastic further reduces strain;
- damage caused by friction when fabric is constantly rubbed between two hard surfaces can be reduced by carefully stitching a thin piece of washable foam on the inside of the garment, eg elbows, seat of trousers, knees. Stitches can be picked up on the inside of a knitted garment and an extra layer of knitting can be worked onto the areas which undergo heavy wear. Leather patches on the elbows of jackets and jerseys may be acceptable for adults and children, and other patches can be a fashion feature on the outside of young children's clothes. Decorative patches on the outside of an adult's garments are usually unacceptable to both the wearer and carer;

## Footwear

Excessive wear and tear on soles and shoe
uppers may be caused by foot irregularities
or abnormal gait. Thicker soles are
generally more durable especially if made
with polyurethane vulcanised rubber or
polyvinyl chloride. Soles repaired regularly
before they become worn will last longer.
Uppers are not so easy to repair and it is
wise to give added protection before
damage occurs. Seams in the upper
construction will weaken the shoe and the
join between sole and upper is another

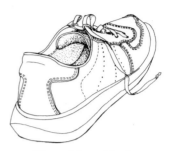

*Shoe with a wider base*

vulnerable area. If the sole and upper are torn apart by a tendency to rock,
then a shoe with a wider base may be the solution. 'Scuff Guard' is a coated
leather that is resistant to scuffing, but since it reduces permeability carers
should check that the wearer's feet are not liable to be too hot and wet.
Other coating solutions can be applied to the areas subjected to the most
wear. Toe caps to prevent scuffing the toe of the shoe can be supplied on
prescription, but they may look unsightly and often fail to protect the
vulnerable area where the upper meets the sole. The Footwear Adviser at
the Disabled Living Foundation can give details of suppliers and the best
method of reinforcing footwear. The appearance of the shoe must always
be considered when looking for ways of reducing wear.

## *Summary: damage to clothing and footwear*

● Carers should look at causes and ways of preventing damage and wear
and tear to clothing.

● Indestructible clothing will not solve the problem of clothing damage if
it is due to inappropriate behaviour.

● Fabric strength depends on the properties of its fibres, how they are spun
into yarns and how that yarn is woven or knitted together.

● Reinforcements to vulnerable points in a garment or shoe can increase
its strength.

● Comfort and the 'look' of the garment must still be considered when
choosing clothes to stand up to excessive wear.

# THE NEED FOR PROTECTIVE CLOTHING

## Drooling

Neuromuscular damage, delayed neuromuscular development or poor muscle control can lead to excessive drooling. Speech therapists, dentists, doctors or psychologists may be able to help in the management of this problem, depending on its cause. If drooling cannot be reduced it will result in stained and damaged clothing, unpleasant odour and persistent dampness, which is uncomfortable, unhealthy and demeaning. Frequent changes of clothing may be a solution but this is time consuming and leads to excessive amounts of laundry. Careful selection or reinforcing of upper garments or making detachable clothing protectors can help to overcome the problems caused by excessive drooling. To ensure that the skin is protected from wetness and to draw attention away from the damp areas, fabric and style are vital considerations whichever of the three methods is used.

## *Fabrics for upper garments and protective panels*

1. 100% cotton or mixes of cotton and synthetic fibres with no less than 75% cotton content will absorb a lot of moisture, and withstand regular washing.
2. Fabrics that are knitted, textured or that have a brushed, looped or pile finish absorb more moisture than smooth surfaced fabrics.
3. Patterned fabrics with an irregular design, multi-coloured or with dark and light shades of the same colour incorporated in the pattern, disguise wet patches better than plain fabrics. If plain fabrics are used, dampness is less obvious on pale than on dark colours.
4. Waterproof backing used when reinforcing garments or when making protective panels should be washable, lightweight, noiseless and micro-porous (ie allow moisture to pass through from the underside). Non-micro-porous waterproof fabric will prevent moisture passing through from the outside, but due to condensation will cause a build-up of moisture from the inside. Specialists in outdoor equipment and garments can supply coated fabrics with these properties, but such fabrics are expensive. A cheaper alternative is water resistant interlining used in the manufacture of rain coats. This interlining is not currently available in the shops but information on possible methods of supply is available from the Clothing Adviser at the Disabled Living Foundation.

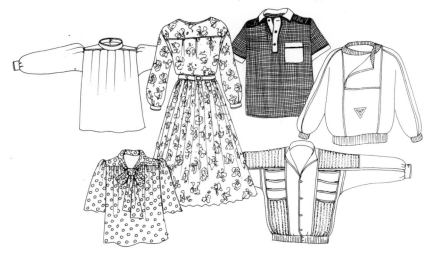

*Garments designed with extra layers of fabric to absorb moisture*

## Styles

*Garments bought 'off-the-peg'*  Upper garments can be bought with more than one layer of absorbent fabric, eg wrap-over collars or front panels, cowl necks, large collars, bows, pleats, gathers and appliqué designs in the area where saliva falls. This extra fabric will absorb and delay the moisture reaching the skin. Fasteners should be positioned away from the area that gets damp and, ideally, it should be possible to remove the garment without pulling it over the head as this can be unpleasant when the garment is wet.

An eye-catching feature elsewhere on the garment will help to draw attention away from the damp areas, eg if saliva falls in the mid-chest area, eye-catching features in the shoulder, neck or sleeve area would be an advantage.

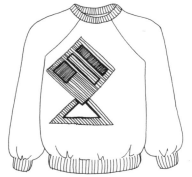

*Reinforcements*  Garments that do not already have built-in features to absorb moisture, can be reinforced by lining front panels or by sewing extra layers of absorbent fabric on the outside, over the potentially damp area; these can take the form of pockets, matching panels or

*Sweatshirt with appliqué design added to absorb moisture*

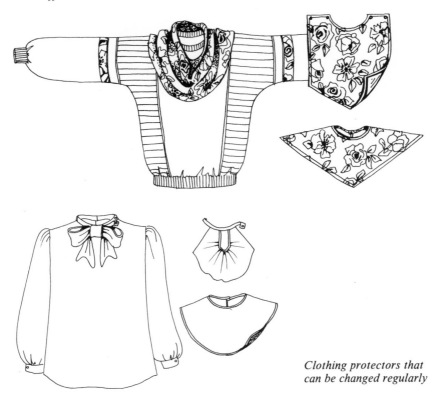

*Clothing protectors that can be changed regularly*

appliqué designs. Water-resistant fabric can be inserted between the inner and outer layers for extra protection. Again, the position of fasteners and the method of removal must be considered to prevent discomfort from dampness when changing. Any extra fabric sewn on the outside must blend in with the overall design and, if possible, the garment should incorporate an eye-catching feature to draw attention away from the damp area.

*Clothing protection* Babies and young children can wear a wide range of bibs to protect their clothes and bodies from dampness caused by drooling, but bibs are inappropriate for older children and adults. The style of clothing protectors made for older children and adults must incorporate certain features; they should: match the individual's chosen style of dress; blend in with other garments worn and not draw attention to the area they are protecting; be of a simple design that is quick and easy to make (because a large number may be needed throughout the day); be designed to protect the appropriate part of the body (eg shoulder, chest); be easy to remove, wash and iron; incorporate fasteners in places where they are unlikely to get wet; and be designed so that it is unnecessary to pull the wet clothing protector over the head. Panels on sweatshirts, collars and scarves are examples of clothing protectors.

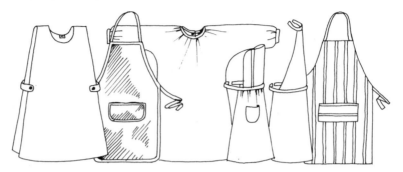

*A wide range of aprons offer varying degrees of protection when eating*

## Food spillage

Eating can be a 'messy' business, especially for someone who is in the process of learning to do so or has some physical or sensory condition that makes feeding difficult. The physiotherapist, occupational therapist and speech therapist may be able to advise on positioning, table height, equipment or eating techniques to reduce this problem. Since it is embarrassing to have spilt food and stains on clothing it is important to find a method of protecting clothing that is not obtrusive or demeaning and is appropriate to the person's age.

A large range of bibs is available for babies and young children but these are inappropriate for older children and adults. A napkin tucked in at the neck is the conventional way of protecting clothing whilst eating; if it will not stay in place, a button hole can be added (or napkins bought with a button hole) in one corner for attachment to a shirt or front-buttoning dress. Napkins made with patterned fabric will be less likely to show stains. However, napkins may not offer sufficient protection.

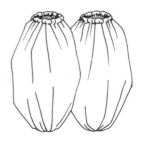

Areas most at risk of staining by spilt food are the front of the garment, the shoulders and the sleeves. A variety of aprons, offering varying degrees of protection, suitable for men and

*Cuff and sleeve protectors*

women of all ages, are available. Tabards or aprons with halter necks cover most of the front of the body; some are clip-on while others require tying or buttoning. Ideally, fabrics should be absorbent and, if spillage is excessive, have a washable or detachable waterproof backing. Those who wish to avoid excessive amounts of laundry can buy PVC aprons that can be wiped clean after each meal or each course. The disadvantage of PVC aprons is that liquid spilt on them will run straight off and possibly onto the bottom of the covered garments. Disposable protective wear can be expensive, is unsightly, and is a potential fire hazard if the wearer smokes.

Sleeves can be rolled up or cuffs turned back during eating to avoid staining, but this may be uncomfortable and interfere with arm movements. Alternatively, cuff and sleeve protectors can be made or bought to be worn while eating. Long-sleeved play coveralls for children give good protection for the front of the body and the sleeves.

## Epilepsy

Some adults and children who have frequent, unpredictable fits, wear helmets to protect them from injury when falling. Bruising may still occur when wearing a helmet, but some carers feel that more severe injury will be prevented by the headgear. When looking at the needs of adults and teenagers, carers should consider the potential risks in the home, school, place of employment, day centre and community, look at the nature and frequency of each individual's fits and find out if these fits can be controlled or predicted, before deciding on a helmet for protection. Helmets do tend to draw attention to the wearer. Protective headgear may encourage the carer to give the person she is looking after more freedom to get involved in daily activities, but she should consider how he looks in a helmet and whether it is detrimental to his integration.

### Style

All protective headgear must be manufactured to British Standard safety specifications and have a secure means of fastening so that it does not fall off during a fit. The helmet should cover the wearer's most vulnerable area – chin, side of head, front of head, back of head – depending on the way he falls.

Carers and wearers may find the wide range of helmets in sports shops for cycling, skateboarding, riding and cricket (conforming to the British Standard specifications for those sports) more acceptable than purpose-made helmets. The Disabled Living Foundation Information Service has lists of commercially available helmets for people who have epileptic fits, and carers should consider the amount of protection given by each helmet, how comfortable it is and how it looks on the individual before deciding on the type to buy.

A consultant can refer someone who has unpredictable fits to the Department of Orthotics for a custom-made helmet. Most regions have access to an orthotist who can make protective headgear which takes account of individual needs and appearance. Remploy are also able to supply made-to-measure headgear.

## Summary: the need for protective clothing

● Carers should look into all other forms of management before seeking a solution through protective clothing.

● The chosen method of protection should cover each individual's vulnerable areas.

● The protective garment should blend in with the wearer's chosen style of dress and not draw attention to problem areas.

● The form of protection chosen should be acceptable to the wearer and carer.

## PHYSICAL FACTORS

### Disproportion

By carefully selecting clothes and accessories, someone with an irregular figure can draw attention to his good points and disguise any irregularities; style, together with the colour and texture of fabrics, can all play a part in this process. There are no strict rules that can be followed as different methods of highlighting and camouflage will work for different people, but bear in mind that the overall appearance must be considered rather than each problem area. Solutions are found by experimenting with style, colour, fabric and accessories.

Apart from the importance of overall appearance, people with unusual proportions may have difficulty finding clothes and footwear that fit well and comfortably. Some large stores stock garments and underwear to fit particular figure types and footwear for short and broad feet or long and thin feet, while other shops specialise in fashion wear for people who are not of 'average' size. Mail order firms offer some specialist services to people with figure and footwear irregularities, and details of stockists can be obtained from the Clothing Adviser at the Disabled Living Foundation. The *Children's Foot Health Register* (available free from: The Administrator, Child Foot Health Register – see Appendix II) lists town and country footwear retailers who stock shoes in four width fittings and provide trained staff to measure the foot. (Donations towards costs are appreciated by both of the above sources of advice.)

People who are not lucky enough to find clothes in the shops or catalogues to suit their needs will have to find other alternatives. Men and women who wear suits may find those that are tailor-made will be worth the expense. Another alternative is to adapt 'off the peg' clothes, or make garments using adapted patterns.

## Adaptations

When buying clothes which may have to be adapted, there are a few points to remember. Since it is easier to 'take-in' than 'let out', always buy a garment that fits the largest dimension; on upper garments make sure that the collar and shoulders fit as well as possible and make the alterations on the rest of the garment; if clothing must be 'let out' make sure there is an adequate seam allowance and that any darts to be 'let out' have not been clipped; the carer should check that any planned alterations will leave the garment hanging correctly. Any reshaping should be done at the side, side/front or side/back seams or darts, leaving the central area at the front and back undisturbed. Several small alterations in different places are often less obvious than one large alteration.

A home dressmaker may be able to alter patterns to suit a particular individual, eg by raising the waistline, increasing width at the hip, decreasing width at the shoulder, while some dressmaking books give instructions on how basic alterations can be made to commercial patterns. Adult education authorities in different areas may run part-time day or evening classes in pattern adaptation; the local library should have details of classes in each area. Once a carer knows how to adapt patterns to suit a particular wearer's needs she can apply the alterations to any commercial pattern to make up a chosen garment.

If no adequate footwear is available to suit an individual's needs, he can be referred through a consultant to a Department of Orthotics where shoes can be adapted or specially made. The shoes will be designed and made to accommodate the individual's foot irregularities, but should also be made in a style and colour chosen by him and should not draw attention to problem areas (see page 111).

(See page 92 for help with sewing and adaptations.)

## Skin problems

Care must be taken when selecting clothing for people who have skin problems; these problems may be due to poor circulation, reduced sensation, allergies, or conditions such as eczema and psoriasis. The aim is to ensure comfort and reduce the risk of skin damage. The carer must be sensitive to any signs of discomfort exhibited by the wearer, especially if he is unable to communicate his needs or unable to adjust his clothing himself, and vulnerable areas of the body should be thoroughly examined daily for any pressure or skin damage. Washing powder may be the cause of skin sensitivity, and carers should find out which brands affect the individual's skin reaction to his clothes.

## Fabrics

Although everyone's needs will be different depending on the cause of their sensitivity, most people prefer the fabric worn next to the skin to be smooth and soft. Natural fibres such as fine cotton and silk will feel comfortable against the skin but some wools and linens may be rough and itchy. Manufacturers of man-made fibres are constantly working to improve the comfort and feel of cloth made from their products to match fabrics containing the best of natural fibres. Stiff fabrics that do not 'give' are uncomfortable especially if the wearer must sit for long periods of time.

## Style

For those with skin problems, clothing should be loose fitting. To avoid pressure sores, creases, folds, rigid seams in jeans, fasteners, pockets and accessories should be avoided at the points where pressure is increased.

Stockings and socks with elasticated tops will restrict circulation if too tight, as will hosiery which is too small. Socks that are very loose will wrinkle and could give rise to pressure sores. Patterns and deep ribbing on socks will also cause uneven pressure and could lead to sores on the skin. Wrinkles can be a problem if tube socks are worn, as the lack of shaping leaves excess fabric in folds at the front of the ankle.

Comfortable shoes are important for everyone, but for those who have poor circulation or poor sensation and are perhaps unable to communicate

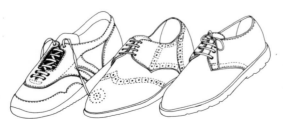

*Shoes with openings allowing easier access to the foot*

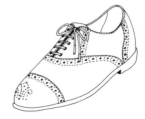

*Oxford-style openings which restrict access*

their needs, the carer must be even more sensitive to their foot comfort. Feet should be checked daily for any reddened pressure areas. Footwear must also be checked for hard seams, protruding nails, wrinkled tongues, stones or irregularities inside the shoe that would lead to rubbing or uneven pressure. When putting shoes onto another person, the carer must make sure that his toes are lying flat; this is made easier if shoes that open to the toe or allow a finger to be inserted to feel the toes are worn. Training shoes are popular and often open as far as the toes, while other conventional shoes with Gibson or Derby styles of apron-fronted lacing allow easy access to the toes. Oxford-style lace-ups are less suitable as they have a 'V'-shaped opening which is more restricting when the shoe is opened up. Information on the specialist range of open-to-toe boots and shoes is available from the Footwear Adviser at the Disabled Living Foundation. Some people may find that this range of open-to-toe shoes and boots does not suit their style of dress and may prefer sandles or fashion shoes with open toes. Whatever style is chosen, consideration must be given to the ease with which foot comfort can be checked and the amount of support the shoe provides when used for walking or when the wearer is merely standing, sitting or transferring to another chair. Some shoes can be adapted to increase access when checking for comfort (details of these adaptations can be obtained from the Disabled Living Foundation).

Since new shoes often cause pressure areas and damage to skin, they should, at first, only be worn for short periods of time, after which feet should be checked thoroughly for pressure areas or soreness.

Further information on fabrics and clothing for people whose skin is sensitive for whatever reason, can be obtained from the National Eczema Society (see Appendix II).

## Control of body temperature

The body's system for regulating temperature is sometimes unbalanced, and this, combined with excessive activity or long periods of inactivity, can give rise to extremes in body temperature which cause discomfort. The effects of changes in room temperature need to be observed by those caring for people who are unable to communicate their needs or adjust their clothing independently; a constant watch should be kept for signs of discomfort. Careful selection of fabric and style can help to maintain a constant body temperature.

### *Perspiration*

Excessive perspiration will lead to odour, discomfort and, possibly, skin damage or irritation if the damp clothes are left in contact with the skin.

*Fabrics*   Cotton, viscose and modal fibres are made up into fabrics that keep the body cool. Thin, smooth yarns do not trap any air inside them and so will feel cool. Loose weaves and open-knit weaves allow air to pass through.

Absorbent fabrics, such as cotton, linen, viscose, rayon, or mixtures of these fabrics, will absorb perspiration, but if worn next to the skin the garment will feel damp.

Fabric made with thin, loosely spun yarns that are woven or knitted loosely will encourage moisture to evaporate so that the garment can dry quickly.

Open weave and loose knitted synthetic fibres, such as 100% polyester, will not absorb perspiration; however, when they are worn next to the skin, moisture will pass through the open weave and can be absorbed by an outer garment made with absorbent fabric so that a dry layer of fabric is left next to the skin. Fabrics made with closely woven, synthetic fibres will trap perspiration next to the skin. There is some debate as to whether or not odour becomes impregnated in synthetic fabrics, particularly polyester, after repeated contact with perspiration; if odour retention in fabric is a problem, perhaps it would be better if those particular synthetics are avoided by the wearer.

As the foot has more sweat glands than any other part of the body it is important to consider ways of reducing the effects of excessive perspiration. Socks made of natural fibres will absorb moisture, but a damp sock is not comfortable. Loosely knitted socks made from synthetic fibres will allow perspiration to pass through and a leather shoe will absorb that moisture – leaving a dry sock against the skin. Synthetic uppers or leather shoes lined with synthetic fabric will not absorb moisture and the perspiring foot will remain uncomfortably damp.

*Styles*   A well fitting, supportive bra made with a fabric that allows moisture to pass through and evaporate may help to prevent sore patches developing under the breasts of a heavily built woman. Men often prefer cotton boxer shorts to close fitting briefs as they have no restricting elastic around the legs. In general, loose fitting styles are preferable because they allow air to circulate between the body and the fabric, removing heat and moisture from the body.

## Poor tolerance of cold

Clothing can maintain body heat but does not produce heat, so the body must be warm before and during dressing. Clothing can also be gently warmed before it is put on. The fact that air trapped in the fabric, between layers of fabric or between the skin and the garment, is responsible for preventing heat loss should be borne in mind when clothes for those who have a poor tolerance of the cold are being selected.

*Fabrics*    The heat retaining properties depend on the make-up of the fabric as well as on the properties of the individual fibres. Wool, polyester and acrylic fibres, which trap air and resist compression, are warm fibres. Thick fabrics, or those which trap air in the surface pile, in the weave or knit, will have an insulating effect, eg terry, quilted and knitted fabrics. As these fabrics get older they tend to become thinner or compressed and lose some of their heat retaining properties. Thermolactyl fibres produce a warmer fabric than others of the same weight and thickness, but require careful laundering and drying to prevent shrinkage. Some shops label clothes as 'Thermal' when they do not contain thermolactyl fibres; this label merely indicates that the garment is thicker and warmer than others in the range.

   Sheepskin and fur are very warm fabrics, but since they are inclined to be heavy and stiff they may make the wearer feel uncomfortable when he is getting dressed and if they are worn for a long time.

   Fabric that is closely woven or showerproofed can be worn as an outer garment over insulating fabrics to decrease the escape of warm, trapped air.

*Styles*    The greater the area of body covered by clothes, the less heat will be lost; long sleeved vests and long johns will therefore help to maintain body heat. Over-garments should fit snugly at neck, waist, wrists and ankles to reduce warm air loss. Accessories, such as scarves and belts, will help to maintain a snug fit. Long sleeved garments will help to keep hands warm, and fingerless mits can be worn indoors without interfering too much with hand function. Textured tights, leg warmers, thick socks or socks with terry or a pile finish on the inside, sheepskin insoles, sheepskin slippers and fur-lined boots will all help to maintain foot warmth. Foot-wear must be large enough to allow trapped air to insulate the foot; tight socks, shoes or boots which exclude air will lead to cold feet.

## Incontinence

This common problem is distressing and causes discomfort and loss of dignity. The reasons for incontinence must be investigated before a clothing solution is sought; a regular toileting routine or toilet training, together with a more careful choice of clothing, may help.

## *Clothes choice when learning to use the toilet*

Those who are participating in a toilet training programme or who require regular toileting or assistance while using the toilet, would benefit from

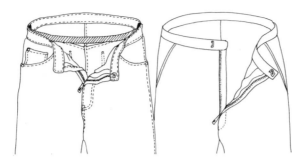

*Adaptations made to trousers to help when learning to use the toilet*

carefully selected clothing that is easy to manage and helps to maintain dignity. Individual preferences must still be considered when clothing choices are made.

*Styles*   Clothing should be kept to the minimum, and since the wearer or carer must be able to manipulate fasteners with ease the type of fastener and its position must be considered.

Separate trousers and tops are more convenient than all-in-one jumpsuits or dungaree designs since only the lower half needs to be removed, leaving the upper part of the body covered. Trousers must be styled so that they are easy to pull down and up again. Men who have difficulty opening their trousers far enough at the front when using the toilet standing up could have their fly fastener extended with a longer zip and underwrap added (underpants would also need an extended opening). Those men who find it easier to open their fly fastener and waistband when standing to use the toilet could have their trousers held up with a piece of elastic sewn on the inside of one side seam, passing across the front of the waist and fastened to the opposite side seam, so that both hands are left free. Women should avoid very full or tight skirts as these will be difficult to lift out of the way quickly when they are learning to use the toilet independently.

*Underwear*   Waist length vests and camisoles are preferable to hip or thigh length styles as they do not get in the way. Pants can be bought in various styles and fabrics and each individual will have their own preference.

## Clothes choice when incontinence persists

If incontinence persists despite efforts to discover the cause and the establishment of a regular toileting routine, a wide range of pads and protective pants is available; the Incontinence Advisory Service at the·

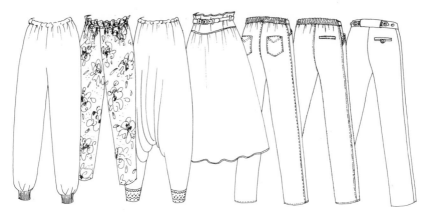

*Full or semi-elasticated waistbands*

Disabled Living Foundation can suggest what would be most suitable and acceptable for each individual.

Bulky pads may affect the fit of trousers and skirts; if there is no suitable, less obtrusive alternative, clothing may have to be bought in a larger size to accommodate these pads. The resulting baggy waistbands will need a belt or elastic inserted to ensure a good fit; short lengths of elastic inserted at each side or at the back of a waistband may look better than a fully elasticated waistband. Waterproof fabric used in pads often crackles and can be embarrassing to the wearer; a pair of cotton pants worn over the protective wear will reduce this crackle when moving about.

Pads will only hold a small amount of urine, and unless they are changed regularly and the wearer is encouraged to use the toilet, accidents will happen, causing discomfort and loss of dignity. The carer will have to cope with regular washing of wet or soiled clothing, although clothes and fabric which may help to minimise these problems can be selected.

*Fabrics*   The textile care label will give details of the fibres included in each garment. Fabrics containing both synthetic and natural fibres will usually withstand frequent washes and, if the laundry instructions are followed, the garments will retain their finish. These fabrics will also require little or no ironing.

Some fabrics will, in time, become impregnated with odours especially if dry cleaned. Thorough washing of the garment as soon as it has become wet or soiled will help to prevent odour retention (see page 94). Synthetic fibres, such as 100% polyester, thought to have odour retaining properties, should perhaps be avoided when selecting pants and lower garments that are frequently wet or soiled. Fabrics with unstable dyes and patterns that will not survive frequent washes and soaking in biological powders should also be avoided.

*Clothing*   Separates, such as skirts/trousers, shirts without tails, half slips, waist length vests or camisoles, are a practical choice for someone who is incontinent, since only lower garments need to be changed. Dresses and nightwear designed to be taken off over the head should be avoided as undressing can be unpleasant if clothing is wet or soiled.

Footwear often becomes wet or soiled. A range of machine washable shoes is available from specialist firms, although some plastic shoes and trainers from ordinary retailers can often be washed satisfactorily.


## Menstruation

A wide range of sanitary pads and tampons, which can be anchored or inserted in a variety of ways, is available. Women and their carers should investigate what is available and experiment to find the most suitable and acceptable method of protection. Factors that must be considered before a choice is made are: the heaviness of the woman's periods, whether or not she could manage them independently, her way of life and style of dress.

Staining, odour and bulky pads showing through tight fitting or flimsy clothes are problems often encountered during menstruation that may affect clothes choice.

Pads will leak through the sides or the bottom if the flow of blood is heavy. When in contact with air, the bacteria in menstrual fluid multiply and, if left, will give rise to an unpleasant odour. Careful selection of underwear and fabrics will not help this problem; the only solution is frequent changes of pads and regular washing. To protect clothes from staining, protective pants designed for those who have incontinence problems can be worn when the flow of blood is heavy but this is an inappropriate and unacceptable solution to most women.

When staining occurs frequently, women should be encouraged (at that time) to wear clothes made of fabrics that stand up to regular washing and stain removing techniques.

Many women will find tampons the most satisfactory form of protection during menstruation, but those who cannot insert tampons independently, who prefer pads or who use pads when their flow is heavy may have to consider what clothes they should wear. Pads vary greatly in shape, size and absorbency and, since the largest pads do not necessarily absorb the most, experimentation is necessary. Those who must wear bulky pads may prefer snug fitting pants to hold the pad in place, but should avoid tightly fitted trousers and skirts.

When learning to manage periods independently, women would be wise to choose styles of dress that can be easily lowered or lifted and held in place when using the toilet, inserting a tampon or attaching a pad. Very full skirts will get in the way and tight fitting skirts and trousers will restrict movement in the toilet. All-in-one jumpsuits and dungarees, for example, may also be a hindrance when this skill is being mastered.

## Wheelchairs and moulded seats

When helping to select clothing for people who spend a large part of their day seated, carers must consider each individual's taste, and offer them a selection of clothing in their chosen style that is easy to get on and off, is comfortable and looks attractive when they are sitting down. Moulded seats are individually fitted to maintain a comfortable or functional position. When making the moulds, technicians should take the thickness of clothing worn into consideration.

## *Underwear*

Front-opening rather than back-opening bras may be easier to manipulate when seated. French knickers and boxer shorts, with no restricting elastic

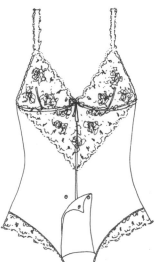

*Cami-knickers with an extended crotch flap*

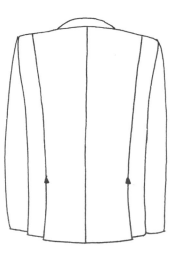

*Jacket with two vents at the back*

around the legs and which allow the air to circulate, are often more
comfortable than close fitting styles for those who sit for long periods.
These loose fitting styles are usually easier to put on and remove while
sitting. Cami-knickers with an opening at the crotch or very wide legged
French knickers may enable the wearer to use the toilet without removing
underwear. The flap on cami knickers can be extended to bring the
fasteners into a more accessible position. Boxer shorts with a button at the
waistband will open wide when the wearer sits to use a urinal bottle and
when he gets dressed and undressed; lengthening the fly opening may also
help (see page 80). Waist length vests and camisoles are more convenient
than longer styles as they do not get in the way. Women may find that
stockings and suspenders rather than tights are easier to put on when
seated; they also have the advantage that they do not have to be removed
when using the toilet.

## Overclothes

People who have to sit when dressing and undressing often find that
separates are easier to put on and take off than all-in-one garments. Tight
fitting skirts and trousers with narrow legs, especially if they are made from
thick cotton or denim, can be uncomfortable for someone who has to sit for
long periods of time; garments made with stretch denim may be a
satisfactory alternative.

Skirts that can be tucked into the waistband when transferring onto a
toilet, and wrap-around skirts that can be left in position on the wheelchair
while the woman sits on the toilet, have the advantage that they leave both
hands free for transferring. Culottes or divided skirts are often chosen by
women whose method of sitting requires them to wear trousers but who
like the look of skirts. Experimenting with the different styles of skirt is the
only way to find out what suits each individual's needs and taste. Trousers
and skirts can be adapted or specially cut to fit the needs of men and women
who have to sit for long periods of time. Details of adaptations and patterns
can be obtained from the Clothing Adviser at the Disabled Living
Foundation. Trousers and skirts bought 'off the peg' should be bought
slightly longer than required as the hemline will ride up when the wearer sits
down. Hems that are altered when the wearer is seated are more likely to
look level. Those who buy suits 'off the peg' will find that a double vent
style will help to ease the jacket over the hips when they are seated; those
who prefer to wear suits may find it worth while to buy a more expensive
suit cut by a tailor to fit their individual needs.

A wide variety of tracksuits is available for both men and women and
many people who use wheelchairs or sit in moulded seats find them easy to
manage and comfortable for everyday wear. Tracksuits, however, are not
suitable for all occasions and do not suit all figures.

Those who are actively involved in transfers or propelling their own wheelchairs will find that gathers, pleats or 'stretchy' fabrics across the back of upper garments give them greater comfort and freedom of movement. Sleeves that have fullness at cuff level should be avoided as they may come into contact with the moving parts of the chair. Cuff protectors can be made in matching fabric to overcome the problem of cuff damage.

Anyone who has to sit for any length of time, especially in a seat that is moulded to fit closely to the body, should make sure that any fasteners, gathers, seams and accessories on garments are not in a position where they will be pressed into contact with the body. The additional pressure caused could lead to sore areas on the skin. Fasteners placed in the centre front position to avoid discomfort may tend to gape. Side front openings on dresses, blouses and skirts often lie better when the wearer is seated. Blouses and shirts can be bought with fasteners at the shoulder or short openings at the centre front of the neck.

## Outdoor wear

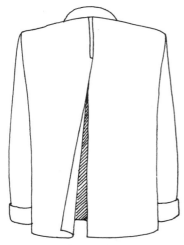

*Opening made in the back seam of a jacket*

Overcoats are a particular problem to people who sit in a moulded seat in their wheelchair. Coats are often too thick to fit into the mould, and if extra space had been allowed when the mould was fitted, the seat would offer inadequate support when the sitter was not wearing the coat. Thinner wind- and water-proof jackets can be worn outside to overcome the problem of space in a fitted seat, but gloves, hats, vests and legwarmers, for example, could also be worn to compensate for the lack of a thick insulating overcoat.

Putting overcoats and jackets on while sitting in a wheelchair or moulded seat is often difficult. Some carers put coats and jackets on back to front. This ensures warmth and easy access to the coat, but looks unacceptable to many wearers. Some women have bought capes that can be worn with the opening at the back, and large capes and ponchos that will cover both the wearer and his moulded seat or wheelchair are available. To make access easier while maintaining the look of the coat or jacket at the front, openings can be added in the back panel. Carers must experiment with different styles to find one that not only suits each particular individual's need for warmth, comfort and style but also allows easy access.

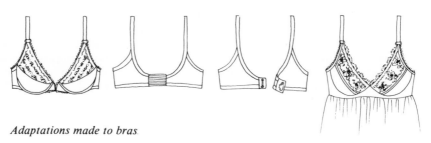

*Adaptations made to bras*

## Limited function in hand and arm

Reduced function in the hands or arms, which may be due to lack of strength or limited range of movement, may lead to difficulties with dressing.

How to choose clothes and fasteners to make dressing easier is discussed on page 56, but some specific problems arise when there is limited hand or arm function.

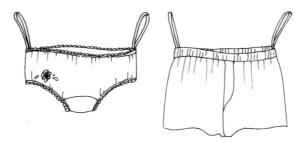

*Loops at each side help when pulling up pants*

### *Underwear*

Small fasteners on bras may be difficult to do up at the back. Some women will find it satisfactory to fasten the bra at the front and move it to the back. The Clothing Adviser at the Disabled Living Foundation can give details of the company which makes a bra with no fastening. Bras with a fastener at the front, which are often easier to manage, are available from many shops. A sales assistant should be able to help anyone who cannot find the type of bra they want and know if front fastening bras are available. Bra slips can be bought without fasteners and may be a satisfactory substitute.

Some adaptations could be made: small hooks could be replaced with larger trouser hooks and bars; a strip of elastic could be sewn in to replace the fastener; and bra slips without fasteners could be shortened to make a camisole top suitable for wearing with trousers. Men and women with a weak grip who find it difficult to pull pants up and down might find it easier if they could pull the pants up with one finger or thumb inserted into loops sewn in at either side of the garment.

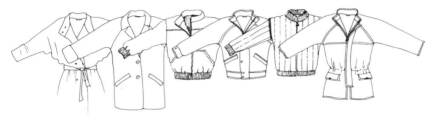

*Coats that may be easier to put on*

## Outdoor wear

A person with limited function in his hands or arms can find it difficult to manage overcoats, which are rarely made with fabric that stretches. Dolman, drop and deep raglan sleeves may make management easier. Some people choose capes because they have no awkward sleeves, while ski jackets with detachable sleeves, which can be eased on separately, have been found suitable for men and women who have fixed joint deformities at their elbow or wrist.

### Summary: physical factors affecting clothes selection

● Carers may have to consider the fibres, fabric make-up and style when selecting clothes to overcome specific physical problems.

● Solutions can often be found by careful selection in shops.

● Those whose needs are not met by local shops may be able to find a specialist mail order company that caters for them, or their clothing may have to be adapted or specially made to suit their needs.

● Carers must remember the importance of each individual choosing his own style of dress.

● When finding a solution to a clothing problem, comfort and the overall appearance of the outfit must always be considered.

# FURTHER READING

Hughes, J. *Footwear and footcare for adults*. London, Disabled Living Foundation, 1983
*Footwear and footcare for disabled children*. London, Disabled Living Foundation, 1982.
(comprehensive practical guides for direct carers on all aspects of footwear, hosiery and maintaining foot health, with sources of further information and assistance)

Turnbull, P and Ruston, R. *Clothes sense: for disabled people of all ages*. London, Disabled Living Foundation, 1973, revised 1985.
(a guide to choosing and adapting clothing for people with physical handicaps)

Lamb, J and Jenkins, G. *FabricWise*. London, Disabled Living Foundation, 1987.
(a guide to the properties of different fabric and how to select fabrics to overcome clothing problems)

McCarthy, B. *Disabled Eve: aids in menstruation*. London, Disabled Living Foundation. 1981. Out of print but may be available in libraries.
(looks at the problems of managing menstruation for women with physical limitations, information on equipment that has been developed)

**Other useful material**

Resource papers from the Disabled Living Foundation:

*Clothing for continence*
*Clothing for people who drool excessively*
*Clothing for wheelchair users*
*Clothing for people with figure irregularities due to scoliosis*
*Footwear*

These and other lists are available for a small charge from: The Disabled Living Foundation, 380-384 Harrow Road, London W9 2HU. Advice and information can also be given over the telephone or by letter to the Clothing Adviser at the above address (tel: 01 289 6111).

# 5

# Caring for clothing and footwear

Looking after your appearance involves maintaining personal hygiene, selecting and caring for appropriate clothing and footwear and checking how you look when you are dressed. This chapter describes how the burden of clothing care can be eased and how the wearer can be encouraged to take more responsibility for his own clothing and overall appearance.

## STORING CLOTHES

When teaching dressing skills and encouraging independent dressing, it is important to have adequate facilities for storing clean and dirty clothes. Each person should have his own cupboard and drawers, so that he knows which clothes are his. The ideal storage facilities allow the wearer easy access to clothing when dressing or undressing, can be divided into separate sections for different clothes so that the wearer can see what clothes he has, and are spacious enough to enable garments to be taken out and put back without disrupting the rest of the clothes and to enable clothes to be hung and folded without crushing. Everyone has their own standards of tidiness and few bedrooms have storage facilities with all the requisites mentioned above, but existing cupboards and drawers can be improved to make them more suitable for someone who is selecting his clothes and footwear each day, while still allowing him to keep the rest of the bedroom as he chooses.

People who live in residential units are often restricted, by fire regulations, to a standard issue wardrobe with drawers which is inadequate for clothing storage. This furniture is often specially made (the Health Service issues type 'C' furniture) to comply with fire regulations. When new furniture is being ordered care staff (through the budget holder and supplies officer) can make recommendations to the manufacturers for special features to be included in the design. If these specifications are requested from the manufacturer at an early stage and for 25 or more pieces of furniture, then the final cost should be little more than the original quote. The size and design regulations issued to manufacturers who supply residential units with furniture can be flexible, eg to give more hanging

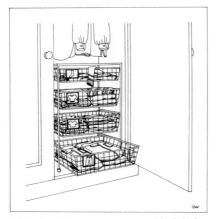

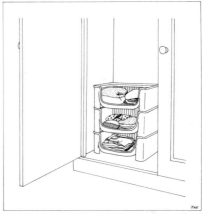

*Wire baskets on runners with labels indicating contents.*

*Stacked vegetable racks can make extra shelves*

space and less drawer space; to supply mirrors (glass or plastic) in any shape or position. The Health Service employs interior design consultants, either attached to a region or within separate districts, who are keen to give advice to carers in residential units about design features that can be incorporated into regulation furniture (these consultants can be contacted by phoning the Regional Health Authority whose number should be in the telephone directory under the name of each region).

## If space is limited

In the home environment, space may be limited and the following ideas may help carers in the home and in residential units to reorganise storage facilities to make choosing clothes easier for each individual:

● store all out-of-season clothes and footwear in storage areas that are less accessible than those allocated for everyday clothes: top shelves, drawers under the bed, in suitcases or boxes on top of the wardrobe or under the bed, in unused cupboard space in another room. The wearer could be involved in putting away summer/winter clothes, both as a learning exercise, and so that he understands that the clothes have only been put away and will be brought back when the season changes;

● laundry baskets should be kept near the bed or in a convenient place so that dirty clothes can be put into it when taken off – taking away any temptation to return them to the wardrobe;

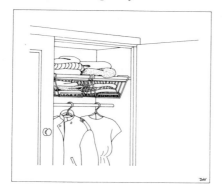

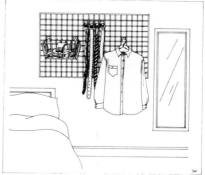

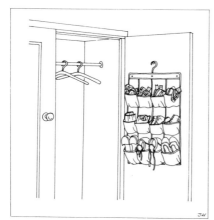

*(above left)*
*Undershelf baskets.*

*(above)*
*Wall grids for hangers and accessories.*

*(left)*
*Shoe tidies used for shoes or clothes*

- extra hanging space is helpful for those who have difficulty folding clothes, shirts and trousers for example, so that they can hang them up instead;
- cupboard and drawer handles can be replaced with larger ones that are easier to use when opening and closing drawers. Centrally positioned drawer handles make opening and closing easier than one handle at each end;
- drawers can be divided by attaching strips of wood with grooves on the front and back inside panels and inserting movable pieces of plywood to divide the space. Wire baskets or plastic containers could be fixed into the drawer to give extra divisions;
- wire baskets on runners in a wire framework can be put into wardrobes to give extra drawers (with or without castors);

- stacked vegetable racks can be put into hanging space to make extra shelves;
- under-shelf baskets can be used to store smaller items, eg underwear, accessories;
- wall grids can be put up in bedrooms with mounted hooks and wall baskets to store smaller items and accessories so that they are clearly visible;
- 'shoe tidies' mounted on coat hangers on cupboard doors can be used to store shoes or smaller articles of clothing;
- strong hooks on bedroom doors or near the front door can be used to store overcoats and outdoor wear.

Carers could look in the bedroom, kitchen and office furniture sections of large stores for ideas for space dividers, or look in local hardware shops, DIY shops and jumble sales for ideas for individual storage needs.


## SEWING AND REPAIRS

When 'off-the-peg' clothes need to be adapted or reinforced, or whole garments must be made, carers need the time, equipment and skills necessary to carry out those tasks. Some carers who do not have those resources will have to look elsewhere for assistance:

- in residential units, staff are sometimes employed in the sewing room to carry out repairs, alterations and reinforcements, and occasionally to make up whole garments for individual residents. It is important that sewing room staff are involved with the carer and resident in planning garments and adaptations so that they are aware of each person's needs and do not make inappropriate or inadequate adaptations. Involvement of the sewing staff at the planning stage may give them more incentive to solve the problem with a garment that meets all the wearer's needs. Sewing staff may also give valuable advice on fabrics, fasteners and styles when making adaptations and complete garments;
- some dry cleaners offer a repair service, and tailors and dressmakers in the community will make up garments and carry out adaptations to individual specifications. These services can be expensive and estimates should be requested before work begins;
- voluntary bodies such as the Women's Royal Voluntary Service (WRVS) have sewing circles, and may take on work to adapt, reinforce and repair clothes or make whole garments. The local WRVS office number can be found in the telephone directory;
- school outfitters may be sponsored by social services or voluntary

bodies to employ tailors and dressmakers to make adaptations to standard school uniforms;

- in some parts of the country parents' self-help groups can offer practical assistance with sewing and repairs (Citizens Advice Bureaux will have details of any groups in the area);

- the Clothing Adviser at the Disabled Living Foundation can give details of the nearest Clothing Workshop, where whole garments can be made to suit the needs of each individual when 'off-the-peg' clothes are not adequate for his needs. The Clothing Adviser can also give general advice on adaptations to garments and patterns;

- local education authorities run part-time dressmaking, pattern adapting and tailoring courses during the day or in the evening, giving carers the opportunity to learn new skills and use the equipment and expertise of the tutors.

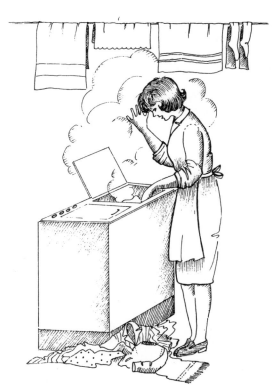

*Washing and drying clothes can be a burden*

# CLEANING CLOTHES

All carers and people who take responsibility for looking after their own
clothes should have some awareness of the different washing processes
suitable for different fabrics. When buying clothes, care labels should be
checked so that the cleaning needs are known before purchase, eg garments
that are likely to become dirty frequently should stand up to regular
washing, whereas clothing for special occasions could be 'dry clean only'.
To obtain a guide to the national textile care labelling symbols write to: The
Home Laundering Consultative Council (see Appendix II).

## Incontinence and drooling

Washing and drying clothes can be a great burden, especially if
incontinence or drooling leads to increased amounts of laundry. All soiled
clothing should be washed separately and should be dealt with within one
day if staining is to be avoided. Urine and saliva will stain and sometimes
leave a lingering odour on clothing that is washed in the conventional
manner; immediate soaking for a few hours, or overnight, in a covered
bucket of cold water with biological powder before washing can help
remove stains and odour. Some people have skin allergies to powerful
biological powders and may find that Napisan, or a similar solution
designed for use with babies' nappies, is just as effective.

In the event of urinary or faecal infection, soiled garments must be
sluiced and washed separately with hypochlorite solution (eg Milton)
added to the final rinse.

## For those who live in the community

Additional help with laundry is available in some areas through district
health authorities and social services departments, and carers should get in
touch with their area office to find out about local facilities. An
incontinence laundry service will deal with all soiled linen and clothing. If
there is no laundry service in your area, assistance is sometimes available
through the home help service.

Automatic washing machines and tumble driers can help to relieve the
burden on carers who wash by hand, in twin tub machines or at the
launderette. Carers may be eligible for financial assistance to buy washing
machines and tumble driers (see page 109 for further information).

## For those who live in institutions

Use of hospital or social service laundries releases carers from the burden of
washing and ironing clothes but may lead to loss of garments and damage

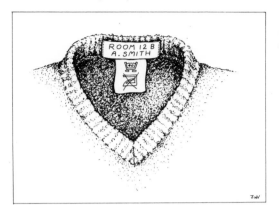

*Clear labels are important to enable residents and care staff to identify clothes*

to clothes made with delicate fabrics. Carers involved with shopping for clothes may have to consider laundry facilities when selecting clothing and look at textile care labels (see page 94) to find a fabric that will stand up to centralised laundry treatment. This consideration will greatly limit the choice of fabrics available to the wearer.

There are ways of overcoming the problems of loss and damage to clothing and of increasing the range of fabrics available to residents who are reliant on a central laundry service:

- by minimising the number of different people dealing with each unit's laundry and by involving the laundry staff in the unit and the people who live there, a more personal service can be achieved;

- careful marking of clothing, giving name of owner and ward or hostel where they live, should reduce loss. The marking label should be in a place where it is obvious to laundry staff but cannot be seen when the garment is being worn. If labels are sewn in, the thread used must match the garment, and if iron-on labels are used care should be taken that they do not affect the hang of the fabric. Clearly printed names, initials or symbols could be used to help each resident identify their own clothes. Important information should be kept to the centre of the label, as the edges of the label may become worn;

- carers could separate all delicate fabrics from the laundry load and wash them by hand, at the launderette or have them dry cleaned;

- residents can be encouraged to learn how to care for their own clothes – by hand washing, washing at the launderette or by visiting the dry cleaners (see page 97);

- the centralised laundry can be used for underwear and nightwear only, while the community or ward/hostel based facilities are used for all other clothes;

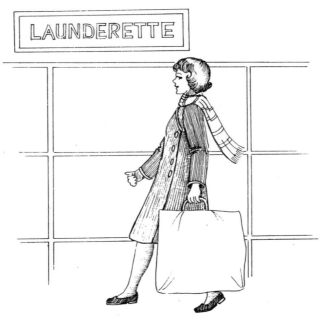

*The local launderette may be a solution*

- domestic or small industrial automatic washing machines can be purchased for use by care staff and residents;
- a tumble drier can reduce the amount of space needed for drying clothes and reduce the need to iron if clothes are folded when the machine is loaded and emptied;

Hostels and other residential units with a limited equipment budget could approach local fund raising organisations for help in purchasing washing machines and tumble driers. If facilities for cleaning delicate garments are unavailable in the central laundry, administrators should be asked if there are any funds available for dry cleaning and the use of launderettes.

## Short term care

Probably because of the turnover of residents and staff and the centralised laundry system, some parents find that clothing is damaged or lost during their child's stay in a local authority or health authority residential unit. Carers in these units advise parents to send clothes that will stand up to a centralised laundry system, that are clearly labelled both with the wearer's name and the unit in which they are staying; they should also make a list of all the clothes sent with the child, keeping a copy for themselves and sending a copy to the residential unit. Carers in the unit should make a list of all the clothes sent with each person, check that they are adequately labelled and keep their list and/or the list sent in by the parents so that they can check that each person returns home with the correct clothing. Carers should approach the administrator of the establishment and claim for any clothing that is lost or damaged.

## LEARNING TO CARE FOR CLOTHES AND FOOTWEAR

The tasks involved in caring for clothes and footwear are: recognising when clothes/shoes need cleaning or repair, understanding which cleaning/repairing process is appropriate, finding a way of getting the cleaning/repairing done – and putting clothes and shoes away again ready for wearing.

Total independence may take a long time to achieve, but any involvement should improve a person's attitude to caring for their clothes and appearance. Involvement can be at any level: it can take place at the school or day centre in a timetabled 'independence training' class; or in the home environment where involvement can be at the appropriate time – each day or once a week, depending on the time available. The level of involvement can vary greatly, depending on each person's ability.

1. Some children and adults will observe the washing or repairing process without taking an active role. It is important that the carer makes the most of this experience by communicating what is happening to each person's clothes and shoes, and why it must be done. The difference between clothes and shoes before and after cleaning or repair should be emphasised so that the wearer will learn to recognise when they need attention.

2. Some people will actively help their carer, eg when clothes are collected for washing, loaded into the machine, washed by hand or taken to the launderette or dry cleaners, ironed and put away, and when shoes are polished or taken to be repaired. This type of involvement will help them to learn the principles of why and how shoes and clothes are cared for and should lead to further involvement.

3. The child or adult who can be taught about the principles and practice of caring for clothes and shoes will be able to take on some of the tasks themselves. The Community Team (see page 55) may be able to give assistance to carers in the home who are starting to teach these skills. Some social service departments employ 'Family Helpers' who will assist in teaching these skills.

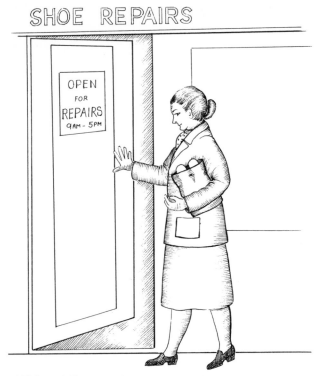

*Taking full responsibility for clothing and footwear care*

4. When all the skills have been learnt, the wearer should be able to take responsibility for caring for his clothes and shoes, at a set time each day or week.
5. Total independence will be achieved when the wearer can take full responsibility for organising washing, cleaning and repair of his own clothes and shoes, can recognise without prompting when it needs to be done, and can organise these chores so that they fit in with his work and social life.

## Teaching guidelines

To teach the practical skills involved in caring for clothes and footwear, the teacher should apply the same techniques outlined in Chapter 1;

*Example X: Ironing 'T' shirt.*

| Name | | |
|---|---|---|
| Date | 22.1.81 | |
| 1. Understands need to iron clothes | I | |
| 2. Erects Ironing Board | P | |
| 3. Plugs iron in | I | |
| 4. Recognises hot and cold parts of iron | I | |
| 5. Understands dangers of hot iron | I | |
| 6. Selects suitable temperature | I | |
| 7. Monitors temperature of iron | I | |
| 8. Spreads 'T' shirt flat on the board | I | |
| 9. Puts iron safely on its end when not in use | I | |
| 10. Irons — front | I | |
| — back | I | |
| — sleeves | I | |
| 11. Checks for creases | V | |
| 12. Folds 'T' shirt | g | |
| 13. Unplugs iron and stores safely | V | |
| 14. Folds ironing board and puts away | P | |

I = Independent
V = Verbal instruction given
g = gestured instruction given
p = physical help given

finding each person's current ability level and progressing step by step from that level, breaking the task down into small stages, providing extra incentives to learn if necessary (see pages 6-15). Examples X (above) and XI (see page 100) show how these tasks can be broken down for different people.

If a person is to be totally independent he must learn, through formal teaching, practice or trial and error – with guidance from the teacher – about the different materials and how they should be cleaned. When first

*Example XI: Using washing machine*

| Name | | |
|---|---|---|
| Date | 15.9.87 | |
| 1. Recognises when clothes need washing | I | |
| 2. Takes clothes from washing basket . | i | |
| 3. Sorts into hot wash and cool wash loads. | V | |
| 4. Opens washing machine door. | P | |
| 5. Loads washing | I | |
| 6. Open soap powder container. | P | |
| 7. Loads correct amount of soap powder. | V | |
| 8. Selects programme. | G | |
| 9. Switches machine on . | G | |
| 10. Recognises when programme is finished. | I | |
| 11. Opens door | P | |
| 12. Unloads washing . | I | |

I = Independent

V = Verbal Instruction

G = Gestured Instruction

P = Physical Help .

learning how to wash, dry and iron different types of fabric, old clothes and large pieces of fabric should, if possible, be used, so that the learner's own clothes are not damaged while the techniques are being mastered.

Everyone has their own method of caring for clothes and shoes, but the teacher may find it an advantage, when passing on these skills to someone else, to look at the equipment used and ways of simplifying the task initially.

## Folding clothes

Start by folding flat square articles, like tea towels, towels and

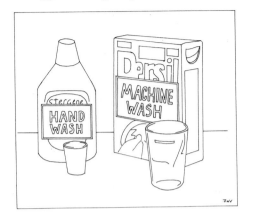

*Clearly labelled containers and measures*

handkerchiefs, and progress to 'T' shirts and jerseys without buttoned openings that can be folded edge to edge.

## Dirty clothes

When removing dirty clothes, always encourage people to turn them the right side out (unless the care label indicates otherwise) before puting into the linen basket; this will prevent tangles when hand or machine washing and make stained areas easier to find (see page 20 for ways of recognising clean and dirty clothes).

## Hand washing and machine washing clothes

When buying clothes, attention should be drawn to the care labels, and those who are able to understand the symbols should be encouraged to check them before washing their clothes. They could also be encouraged to divide up the washing load into categories, eg delicates, light colours, heavily soiled. Wall charts may be useful to some people, linking the care label symbols with the washing programme or technique. Before someone washes clothes by hand, he should be made aware of the areas that will need extra attention, eg armpits, jersey fronts, cuffs and collars, crotch areas, the bottom edge of trouser hems. Use two washing solutions/powders only – one for hand washing and one for machine washing, preferably in different shaped containers (bottle or box) and clearly labelled. Have a measure for each solution/powder showing exactly how much of each is needed for a sinkful of water and one load in the machine. Choose a machine with

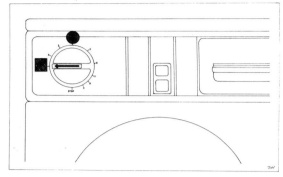 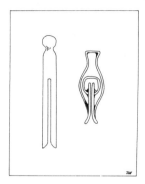

*One or two washing programmes can be labelled*          *Push-on pegs*

simple controls that are clearly marked (colour coded or picture codes are preferable to written codes) or mark with colours or symbols the two or three most commonly used cycles. When unloading the machine, garments should be pulled out individually and placed folded into a laundry basket so that they are easier to sort when drying.

### Tumble drier

Again choose a machine with simple controls. If clothes placed in a tumble drier are folded they will require less ironing when dry.

### Hanging clothes on the line

Two-pronged 'push-on' pegs are easier to manage than clip-on pegs. Clothes that have been folded after being taken out of the washing machine will be easier to hang up, as they won't be tangled. When learning how to peg clothes on the line it is often better to start with small square flat articles, like tea towels and handkerchiefs, and progress to larger more awkwardly shaped garments, like trousers, shirts and dresses. Folding dry garments as they come off the line will reduce the need for ironing.

### Ironing

Accidental contact with an iron can easily burn the skin; before being taught the ironing technique the learner must therefore understand which parts of the iron get hot, how to turn the temperature down or the iron off, how and where to leave the hot iron on the board when not in use, and how to avoid burning fabrics.

For teaching purposes, an iron with simple, clearly visible controls or controls that can be labelled to show hot, warm and cool settings, would be an advantage. The handle must be designed to insulate the hand and keep all hot areas as far away as possible from the hand of the person ironing. If possible, choose an iron which shows clearly, by colour, which parts do not get hot and can be touched, and which parts must not be touched.

When starting to teach the ironing technique, use a warm iron on squares of thin fabrics that iron easily, so that, while the risk of burning is reduced, the learner can see which parts of the iron produce heat and the difference between ironed and unironed fabric. Gradually develop this skill, and, as awareness of danger and understanding of the technique increases, increase the temperature gradually, using thicker fabrics and more complicated shapes, eg trousers, shirts.

Ironing boards are difficult to erect and, before purchasing a new one, it is wise to try to fold and unfold it. If space allows it may be easier to leave the board ready for use.

## Shoe care

Leather uppers need regular polishing if they are to maintain their suppleness and water resistance. The wearer could be encouraged to polish his own shoes at a set time each week to ensure that they are cleaned regularly. An old pair of gloves will help to keep his hands clean while polishing. Some people find it easier to polish shoes with a soft cloth, but if brushes are to be used they can be marked with different coloured labels for use with different shoe colours. The instant and easy-to-apply shoe shining products now available enable more people to take responsibility for cleaning their shoes; however, these solutions do not have the same protective qualities as traditional polish.

Shoes absorb moisture when worn so the wearer could be encouraged to change his shoes once a day by having one pair of outdoor and one pair of indoor shoes, or one pair of day and one pair of evening shoes. Regular changes will enable each pair of shoes to dry out, ensure that foot health is maintained and prolong the life of the shoes. Remember that leather shoes should not be dried out by direct heat.

# CARING FOR APPEARANCE

As well as being taught all the complex skills involved in selecting clothes and putting them on, everyone should be taught to check their appearance. Each person has different standards of dress, and individual choice of style must be respected. It is, however, important that an individual's appearance and personal hygiene does not impede their integration or interfere with their involvement in social and recreational activities. For this reason it is important to encourage people to be aware of their appearance and the impression they give to others.

Checking appearance involves looking at hair style, checking that clothes, hair and body are clean, checking that clothing does not need repair, is worn in the correct order with all the fasteners done up, is pulled straight and is tucked in if necessary. The carer must encourage each person to check his appearance independently and correct any faults himself.

When teaching this skill:

● make sure the learner understands what the carer is expecting him to do;

● make sure there is a mirror (full length if possible) in a well lit, accessible position each morning;

● draw the learner's attention to the need to check appearance and encourage him to do so by looking, feeling and smelling hair, body and clothing. This is more valuable than the carer making corrections for the learner;

● make sure the wearer can see, feel and smell the difference between clothing and appearance before and after correcting them;

● provide verbal or visual clues to remind people of the areas to check each day; for example, a pictorial sequence showing hair, collar, shirt tails and buttons; taped verbal clues (the learner often responds better if his own voice is used on the taped reminder) of the areas to check. These clues should be withdrawn as the skill is learnt.

Some people have all the skills necessary to check and make the most of their appearance, but are not motivated to do so. Carers must try to find out why a particular person lacks motivation and find a way of motivating him.

For example the carer could:

● make him aware of the reasons why appearance and personal hygiene is important, eg he can't go to the shops if his flies are undone; if he smells unpleasant, fewer people will want to spend time with him;

● establish a routine in which a set time each day is allocated for each person to check his appearance and personal hygiene, eg before breakfast, before attending work, day centre or school;

● provide incentives (see page 12) to encourage him to take more care of his appearance and personal hygiene. These incentives should be withdrawn gradually as this skill becomes part of everyday life. Photographs taken when he looks presentable can be a useful incentive to check appearance. When he consistently checks his appearance the incentive can be toned down; for example, by pasting the photos taken previously into an album; by framing the best photo and putting it on the bedroom wall; by looking at photos taken previously and discussing how good he can look. The aim is to increase his motivation to look presentable, and carers should not introduce an incentive without working out how it can be withdrawn without stopping the activity it was rewarding;

• verbal praise from carers, teachers, instructors and friends is a valuable incentive to someone to make himself presentable, and this should continue once the person has learnt to check his own appearance.

## *Summary*

• Careful organisation of clothing storage can facilitate selection of appropriate clothes each day when dressing.

• Carers should look to the community, health service, social services and their own resources to ensure that all clothing and footwear care is completed in a way that suits each wearer's needs.

• Involving the wearer at any level when caring for clothing and footwear is valuable to increase his awareness of the need for these processes.

• Teaching these skills can be approached in the same way as teaching dressing skills, but some consideration could be given to the equipment used and the possible dangers attached to using that equipment.

• Each individual has different standards of appearance, but people should be encouraged to be aware of the effect of their appearance.

• Whether failure to care for appearance is due to lack of knowledge or lack of motivation, each person should be encouraged to check his own appearance rather than having corrections made for him.

## FURTHER READING

Carruthers, C. *Personal care: a lifeskills manual.* Bicester, Winslow Press, 1987.

(a practical guide to carers and professionals involved in teaching advanced independence training, giving information on all aspects of personal care and techniques that can be used to pass on this knowledge to men and women. It includes sections about clothing, appearance and clothing care)

## Other useful material

*A guide to the textile care labelling code.* Available from: The Home Laundering Consultative Council, 7 Swallow Place, Oxford Circus, London W1R 7AA (tel: 01 408 0020)

*Dressing matters.* Disabled Living Foundation, 1987.
Video – for sale
Available from: The Disabled Living Foundation, 380-384 Harrow Road, London W9 2HU (tel: 01 289 6111), and Haigh and Hochland, The Precinct Centre, Oxford Road, Manchester M13 9QA (tel: 061 273 4156).

(a video to teach the viewer about the importance of clothes and to stimulate an interest in style and individuality in clothing worn. Made for adults, using the minimum of speech and text to get the message across)

## Personalised clothing systems

Advice can be given over the telephone or by letter, by the Clothing Adviser at the Disabled Living Foundation (see address and telephone number above) about setting up a personalised clothing system and overcoming the problems of using a centralised laundry service.

# 6

# Financial assistance

An adequate supply of clothes and footwear can be expensive, and people with special footwear or clothing needs, or who generate excessive amounts of laundry or repair work, often cannot meet the cost out of their own, or their carer's, income and resources.

The help available to people with special clothing needs changes periodically and will vary according to the area in which they live. Although this chapter gives general facts about the range of possible practical and financial assistance, each person should seek up-to-date information of the help available in his particular area, and find out how to make the maximum use of these facilities to meet his individual needs. The best sources of free information are locally based and the contacts listed below may be useful.

## SOURCES OF ADVICE

The address and telephone number of the local Citizen's Advice Bureau, which can answer enquiries at the office, over the phone or, occasionally, by making a home visit, can be found in the telephone directory. The Bureaux hold information on the local financial and practical assistance that is available through the DHSS, social services or voluntary organsiations.

Social service area offices (social work departments in Scotland) can provide information on financial and practical problems. Some areas employ welfare rights officers who will advise and help individuals to claim the grants to which they are entitled. The telephone number of each area office can be found in the telephone directory under the name of the local county or borough. The area office will be able to put an inquirer through to the department that can help.

The leaflets published by the Department of Health and Social Security on the financial assistance available can be found in social security offices and some post offices. Addresses of local social security offices are listed in the telephone directory under 'Health and Social Security, Department of'.

In addition, a Freephone service, which can be obtained by dialling 100 and asking for 'Freephone DHSS', gives information on the benefits available; this is an information service only and its advisers are not able to take action on your behalf.

The Disability Alliance (see Appendix II), publishes the *Disability Rights Handbook* (available at a small charge), which explores all the grants available and gives details about how to apply and make the best use of them.

Any advice on local practical help with clothing and footwear care and supply should be sought through the local general practitioner, district nurse, social worker, health visitor or community team (see page 55).

See also Appendix II for addresses of voluntary organisations which give advice or practical assistance.

## Advice for people living in residential units

A resident in local authority or health service accommodation is still entitled to some benefits and allowances that can add to his quality of life. The local authority has a responsibility to provide accommodation and pay for food, clothing and footwear; a minimum charge is made for this service and taken from each person's income at source. Each individual then receives a small personal allowance from their income to cover incidental daily expenses such as entertainment and gifts.

Research carried out by Disability Alliance (1986, Bradshaw and Davis, *Not a penny to call my own*) looks at ways of improving residents' financial independence and the opportunities they have to spend their money as they choose. Greater financial freedom allows people choice in their style of dress; the personal allowance is not intended, and is inadequate, for this purpose. Bradshaw and Davis suggest that: funds allocated in the main budget for clothing in the residential unit should be available as cash for each individual to select and buy his own clothing and footwear; information should be readily available to residents and their carers about benefits and allowances; residents should be encouraged to claim for the money they are entitled to; and if residents choose to put their money in a savings account, the system of deposit and withdrawal should be reviewed regularly so that the money is secure but easily accessible when it is needed.

Because of low staffing levels, residents who need assistance to withdraw and spend their own money do not get the help they need; the resulting accumulated savings in personal accounts will affect benefit entitlement and could lead to a drop in income. Low staffing levels may also make it difficult for each person to buy clothes and footwear with allocated clothing cash at the shops of their choice; but these problems could be overcome if carefully chosen volunteer advocates (see pages 53 and 55) or external appointees (relatives or friends) willing to help residents spend their money as they choose, are utilised.

Staff in residential units who are concerned about the finances of residents should discuss the matter with the budget holder, who may be the Unit Manager, the Nursing Officer or the Officer in Charge. The budget holder, the resident, or a carer who has been made responsible for that resident's finances can seek advice from all the other channels mentioned previously to ensure that each individual is receiving the income to which he is entitled.

See also Appendix II for addresses of voluntary bodies who may give help and advice.


# ALLOWANCES AND GRANTS

People living in the community and in residential units will find that they can claim grants that may help to ease the financial burden of clothing care and supply – some are specifically for this purpose, while others can be used for necessary clothing and footwear.


## Attendance Allowance

This is a tax-free, non-means-tested allowance for anyone aged 2 years or over who needs a lot of looking after at home; it may also be available to people living in health or local authority accommodation who go home on leave. It can be paid at the same time as all other benefits. The allowance, which is intended to make it easier for the disabled person to obtain the care he needs, can be spent on, for example, household expenses, payment for services or to purchase essential items.


## Invalid Care Allowance

This tax-free and non-means-tested allowance can be claimed by a carer who, because she is looking after someone at home, is unavailable for full-time employment. Receipt of Invalid Care Allowance is income for the carer and may affect other benefits claimed at the same time.


## Mobility Allowance

A tax-free, non-means-tested cash benefit paid weekly without affecting other allowances or benefits, can be claimed in full by people living in the community or in health service, local authority, charitable or private accommodation; it is designed to help people with mobility problems to get out of their homes and travel more easily. Once a person has qualified for Mobility Allowance the money can be spent in any way he chooses, eg on extra outdoor clothes, new clothing and footwear for going on outings and holidays, and on paying fares for shopping trips. Mobility Allowance cannot be counted as income and therefore cannot be used as a contribution towards basic living costs in residential units; this makes the Allowance a valuable addition to the personal allowance.

## Severe Disablement Allowance

This is a tax-free, non-means-tested weekly cash benefit for those who are aged 16 years or over, have been incapable of work for at least 28 weeks, and who do not qualify for sickness or invalidity benefit because they have not paid National Insurance Contributions. Anyone receiving Severe Disablement Allowance can still qualify for Attendance Allowance and Mobility Allowance. This allowance can be claimed by someone living in the community or in a residential unit, but will be reduced when he moves into local authority or health service accommodation as his basic living needs are met by the authority.

Other financial assistance for those with a low income or special needs may be available from the Department of Health and Social Security in the form of weekly additions to income or a one-off grant or loan for special equipment, eg a washing machine. The legislation determining the availability of these benefits changes from time to time, and up-to-date information on possible sources of assistance should be requested from the organisations mentioned at the beginning of this chapter (see page 107).

## Family Fund

This fund, run by the Joseph Rowntree Memorial Trust with support from the Government, is available to families caring for children under 16 years who have physical handicaps or severe learning difficulties. The grants given are to complement rather than replace help available from local authorities. A family applying for help from the Fund will be visited by a social worker who will assess the family's eligibility for assistance, taking its financial circumstances into consideration. Families can apply and ask for whatever equipment they need, including a washing machine, tumble drier, clothing (but not school uniform) for children whose clothes wear out quickly or who have special clothing needs, or sewing equipment for carers who wish to make or repair clothes to overcome specific problems.

## Financial help for footwear

A hospital consultant can prescribe specially made or ready-made surgical shoes to overcome foot problems. These shoes are paid for by the National Health Service (NHS) and each eligible person is entitled to two pairs initially, and a further pair every year. Some people, especially children whose feet are growing or people whose shoes undergo excessive wear and tear, may find one pair per year insufficient to meet their needs. In these exceptional circumstances the consultant may agree to prescribe more than one pair of shoes per year. In the case of someone whose foot problem is unlikely to change, the consultant may stabilise his prescription for each pair of shoes for the following five years, so that the shoes can be ordered through the NHS each year without assessment by the consultant. If the consultant feels that the person's footwear needs will gradually change, then each yearly order for shoes must be preceded by a consultant's assessment. If an assessment of footwear needs is carried out by other professionals the shoes will have to be paid for by the wearer; a prescription for surgical shoes must be confirmed by a consultant before they can be paid for and supplied by the NHS. Shoe repair for special shoes will be paid for and carried out by the NHS contractor who made the shoes, but this may take time and any minor repairs that do not affect the special features of the shoe can be taken to the local shoe repair shop and paid for by the wearer. These principles apply to anyone with severe foot problems living at home or in residential units who requires special footwear.

## Schools

### Day schools

Some education authorities will give a clothing allowance to families with a low income to help them buy school uniform, including shoes and sports clothes. The allowance, paid at intervals throughout the child's school education, usually takes the form of vouchers that can be exchanged in certain shops.

### Residential schools

Schools run by local authorities have a fixed clothing allowance every year for each residential pupil. This rate is the same for all schools despite the increased needs of some students with special clothing problems. A supplementary allowance is sometimes available if the average reasonable expenditure after six months supports the claim. The annual allowance is to cover each student's needs while at school, including clothing for sports, outings and social activities. The clothing bought remains the property of the authority and is not for home use. Students travel to and from home in their own clothes. Authorities expect clothes to be ordered through their supplies department, but specialist items can be ordered from other sources via the supplies department. Many schools involve pupils in the choice and purchase or their own clothes and footwear. The education authority can issue a list of recommended local retailers where clothing and footwear can be purchased. Clothing and footwear bought at those local shops can be paid for in cash from the annual allowance; receipts must be kept with a complete record of all the money spent.

## Summary

● Everyone's clothing needs are different and some people find that supplying and caring for clothing is very expensive.

● Financial and practical assistance with clothing and footwear supply and care is available from the DHSS, the health authority, voluntary organisations and the local authority.

● People living at home or in residential units (or their carers) should make enquiries to find out what help they are entitled to and how to make the best use of any money they receive.

● Additional financial assistance may give individuals with special needs, living at home and in residential units, the freedom to choose and buy their own clothes and express their own individuality.

## FURTHER READING

Bradshaw, M and Davis A. *Not a penny to call my own: poverty amongst residents in longstay mental handicap and mental illness hospitals*. London, Disability Alliance, 1986.

(research into the state of patients' finances in institutions and ideas about how staff, relatives and managers can help to resolve the current situation)

Fitzherbert, L and Bellofatto, H *ed. A guide to grants for individuals in need.* London, The Directory for Social Change, 1987.

(provides a comprehensive list of charitable funds available nationally and in specific areas of the country, with information about types of funding and methods of application for grants)

*Disability rights handbook. 1987/8.* London, Disability Alliance. Available from: 25 Denmark Street, London WC2H 8NJ (tel: 01 240 0806)

(a guide to grants available and how to claim them)

# Appendix I: Improving dressing skills: additional activities

The best way to learn dressing skills is to practise them every time clothing is put on or taken off. However, the skills associated with dressing can also be practised at other times during the day when there may be more time for exploration and experiments. All the activities should be appropriate to each person's age and ability, and have an end result or a purpose.

For example:

- understanding of body parts, clothing, colours, textures, and the concepts of over and under, in and out, on and off, could be improved through songs, games, puzzles, painting, collages and movement groups;

- physical activities for the whole body or involving different body parts can improve balance and co-ordination when getting dressed;

- activities undertaken during the day at school or in a day centre, or in the evenings, can be used to build up a person's capacity to concentrate and follow instructions to complete a task;

- some games can be bought or made to encourage the skills needed to manipulate fasteners, eg threading, posting shapes into slots in boxes;

- individual and group activities can improve awareness of appearance if the people taking part talk about and look at themselves and other people in the group, on the TV, when out shopping etc (see page 49);

- domestic skills, such as washing clothes, sorting laundry, hanging out clothes, tidying wardrobes, can all be used as a vehicle for teaching someone about the variation in textures and the different types of clothes (see pages 97-103);

- dressing-up games (for children) and activities that require aprons and overalls can provide the opportunity to experiment more freely with putting on and taking off clothes;

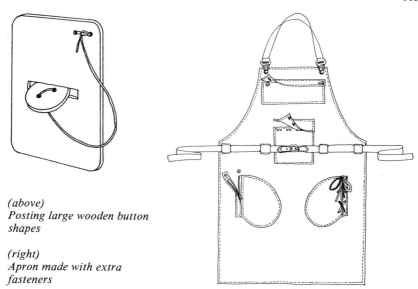

*(above)*
*Posting large wooden button*
*shapes*

*(right)*
*Apron made with extra*
*fasteners*

- opportunities to practise manipulating fasteners may need to be found. Children can practise on dolls clothes, but this is inappropriate for teenagers and adults. Aprons and overalls used for cooking or art activities can, for example, be made with pockets and belts with a variety of fasteners. The ability to manipulate these fasteners can be taught, initially, on a table-top where they are accessible and visible and, once the basic technique has been learnt, the apron/overall can be put on and fasteners manipulated in a less visible and accessible position against the body. Rewards could be put into the pockets as an incentive to practise this skill;

- outdoor coats and cardigans often have larger fasteners than indoor clothes, and the wearer can practise fastening and unfastening every time he goes out or returns;

- some computer programmes have been devised to assess and teach body awareness, sequencing, and placing of clothes. Using the computer can often be a useful incentive for children and adults who are learning these skills. Further information can be obtained from the Research Officer in the Use of Microtechnology with People Who Have Profound and Moderate Handicaps, Special Care Unit at Leavesden Hospital (see Appendix II for the address).

# Appendix II: Useful addresses

The addresses of specialist groups who can give information, advice and, in some cases, practical assistance to carers in the community and in institutions are set out below. The national offices of large organisations may be able to provide local contacts who can give more practical assistance.

*Advocacy Alliance*, 2 St Pauls Road, London N1 2QR (tel: 01 359 8289)

*The Campaign for People with Mental Handicap*, 12a Maddox Street, London W1R 9PL (tel: 01 491 0727)

*Child Foot Health Register*, 84-88 Great Eastern Street, London EC2A 3ED

*Disabled Living Foundation*, 380-384 Harrow Road, London W9 2HU (tel: 01 289 6111)

*Disability Alliance*, 25 Denmark Street, London WC2H 8NJ (tel: 01 240 0806)

*Downs Syndrome Association*, 12-13 Clapham Common Southside, London SW4 7AA (tel: 01 720 0008)

*Family Fund*, PO Box 50, York YO1 1UY (tel: 0904 21115)

*The Home Laundering Consultative Council*, 7 Swallow Place, Oxford Circus, London W1R 7AA (tel: 01 408 0020)

*KIDS for families with children with special needs*, 80 Waynflete Square, London W10 6UD (tel: 01 969 2817)

*Leavesden Hospital*, Watford, Herts WD5 0NU (tel: 0923 674090)

*Makaton Vocabulary Development Project*, c/o Mrs Margaret Walker, 31 Firwood Drive, Camberley, Surrey GU15 3QD (tel: 0276 61390)

*MENCAP National Centre*, 123 Golden Lane, London EC1Y 0RT (tel: 01 253 9433)

*The National Advisory Unit for Community Transport*, Tavistock House North, Tavistock Square, London WC1H 9AX (tel: 01 388 6542)

*The National Autistic Society*, 276 Willesden Lane, London NW2 5RB (tel: 01 451 3844)

*National Eczema Society*, Tavistock House North, Tavistock Square, London WC1H 9JL (tel: 01 388 4097)

*One to One*, Contacts for People with Learning Difficulties, c/o The Director (Mrs J E Willson), 33 Cornelia Street, London N7 8BA (tel: 01 607 8327)

*Royal National Institute for the Blind*, 224 Great Portland Street, London W1N 6AA (tel: 01 388 1266)

*Royal National Institute for the Deaf*, 105 Gower Street, London WC1E 6AH (tel: 01 387 8033)

*Scottish Society for the Mentally Handicapped* 13 Elmbank Street, Glasgow G2 4QA (tel: 041 226 4541)

*SENSE, The National Deaf, Blind and Rubella Association*, 311 Grays Inn Road, London WC1X 8PT (tel: 01 278 1000)

*The Volunteer Centre UK*, 29 Lower Kings Road, Berkhamsted, Herts HP4 2AB (tel: 04427 73311)

# INDEX

activity, and choice of clothing, 18, 19
adaptations of clothing, 75, 92
allowances and grants, 109
appearance check by visually
        handicapped, 31
    checking, 103
apron, protective, 72
arm, reduced function, 86
arrangement of clothes to assist
        dressing, 16
assessment of dressing skills, 1, 6-7
Attendance Allowance, 109
attention difficulties, 39

body awareness, 44
body temperature control, 77-79
boots, *see* footwear.
bras, adaptations, 86
buttons, 58

caring for clothing and footwear,
        89-103
*Children's Foot Health Register*, 74
choice of clothes, *see* clothes, choice.
clean clothes, distinction from dirty,
        20, 31
cleaning, 94-103
clothes, adaptation, 92
    care, 89-103
    care labels, 94, 101
    choice, factors influencing, 64-88
        for activity, 18, 19
        for weather, 18, 19
        in damage due to excessive
                wear and tear, 64
        in damage due to inappropriate
                behaviour, 64
        in gross physical limitations, 74

clean and dirty, distinction
        between, 20
cleaning, 94-103
for easy dressing, 56
    fasteners, 57, 59
    styles, 56
for visually handicapped, 26, 28
order for wearing, 16
personalised system, 106
protective, 69-74
quantity and suitability, 6
reinforcements, 67, 70
repair, 92, 97
selection, 49-63
    age-appropriate, 52
    assistance by storing method,
        17, 89-92
    choice encouragement, 49
    communication difficulties, 51
    guidance, 51
    inappropriate, 52
    safe, 62
    transport to shops, 54
storage, *see* storage.
clothes-pegs, 102
cold, poor tolerance to, 78
communication difficulties, 32-35
    with learner with limited hearing
        and vision, 36
community teams, 55
concentration difficulties, 39
co-operation lack, 44

damage to clothes due to excessive
        wear and tear, 64, 67
    due to inappropriate behaviour,
        64
delayed development, and dressing
        skills, 23

denim, 65, 66
dirty clothes, distinction from clean,
    20, 31
disproportion, physical, clothes for,
    74
dressing,
    environment, 1; *see* environment
    skills, activities for improvement,
        114
        assessment, 1, 6-7
        teaching, guidelines, 1-22, 114
            methods, 10-12
            overcoming additional
                problems, 23-
                48
        time taken, 4
drooling and clothes cleaning, 94
    protective clothing, 69

environment for dressing, 1
    and physical limitations, 24
    and lack of co-operation, 45
    and communication difficulties,
        33
    and perceptual problems, 43
    and visual impairment, 29
    in limited hearing and visual
        capacity, 36
epilepsy, protective clothing, 73
eyesight, impaired, 26-32; *see* visual
    impairment.

fabrics, absorbent, 78
    as aids to dressing, 27, 57
    durability, 65
    heat-retaining, 79
Family Fund (Joseph Rowntree
        Memorial Trust), 110
fasteners, 57-61
financial assistance, 107-113
folding clothes, 100
food spillage, protective clothing, 72
footwear, care, 89-100, 103
    choice for easy dressing and foot
        health, 60-62, 68
    damage due to excessive wear and
        tear, 64, 68
    fasteners, 61
    financial help towards purchase
        and repair, 111

for foot irregularities, 74
for skin problems, 77
for incontinence, 82
for visually handicapped, 28
materials for, 62
reinforcement, 68
storage, 90

grants towards clothing costs, 109
guidance, for visually handicapped,
    30
    for dual sensory impairment, 36

hand, reduced function, 86
headgear, protective, 73
heat loss, 78, 79
hook and eye clothing fasteners, 59

incentives, 12
    for auditory and visually impaired,
        38
incontinence, 79-82
    clothes choice in, 80, 81
    clothes cleaning, 94
Invalid Care Allowance, 109
ironing of clothes, 99, 102

labelling of clothes, 95
laundry service, 94, 96
learner, assessment, 1, 6-7
lifting for dressing, 25

marking clothing, 95
menstruation, protection during, 82
methods of teaching dressing skills,
    6-22, 114
Mobility Allowance, 109

napkins, 72

order of wearing clothes, 16
overcoats, 84, 87

perceptual problems, 42-44
    teaching methods, 43
perspiration, excessive, 77
physical disproportion, clothes for, 74
    limitations, and teaching dressing,
        24
position for dressing, 24

privacy during dressing and
        undressing, 21
progress recording, 7-12, 14
    in visually handicapped, 34, 37
protective clothing, need for, 69-74
    styles, 70

records of progress in dressing skills,
        6-10, 14
    in visual and hearing-handicapped
        learner, 37
repairs, 92, 97
rewards for dressing skills, 12

safe clothing, selection, 62
sanitary pads, 82
school uniform, 111
schoolchildren, clothing allowance,
        111
seats, moulded, clothes for users,
        83-86
selection, *see* clothes, selection
Severe Disablement Allowance, 110
sewing, 92
shoes, *see* footwear
shopping, 54-56
skin problems, suitable clothing, 75
smell to identify clean and dirty
        clothing, 20, 31
storage of clothes, 2, 89
    for learners with perceptual
        difficulties, 42
    for visually handicapped, 28
    method to assist selection, 17
symbols in instruction, 34

teaching other skills necessary for
        dressing and undressing,
        16-21

time in relation to dressing, 4, 5
timing of dressing, 25, 30, 33, 36, 39,
        43, 45
toilet training, 79
transport for shopping, 54
tumble drier, 102

undressing, 7
underwear for people with
        continence problems, 80
    for wheelchair users, 83
    in reduced hand and arm
        function, 86

velcro clothing fastener, 59
    shoe fastener, 61
visual cues in communication, 34
visual impairment, 26-32
    clothing identification in, 30
    dressing environment, 29, 36
    footwear in, 28
    guidance in dressing, 30,
    positioning of clothes, 31
    selection of clothes, 26
    storage of clothes, 28
    teaching methods in, 24
voluntary bodies, help with
        shopping, 55

wardrobe arrangement, 5, 89
    design, 89
    weather and choice of clothing,
        18, 19
wheelchair users, clothing for, 83-86
Women's Royal Voluntary Service, 56

zip fasteners, 58

Printed by Drogher Press, Unit 4 Airfield Way, Christchurch, Dorset, England.